Hair Therapy Presents

A COMPLETE GUIDE TO

Healthy Hair
growth

I0541548

By Cyre' Marie

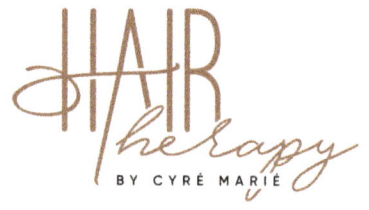

A Complete Guide to Healthy Hair Growth

The Hair Bible: DIY Treatments, Growth Secrets & a Journal for Your Best Hair Yet

An Imprint of Cyre' Marie & Co
Los Angeles, California

First Cyre' Marie & Co edition: March 2025

Cyre' Marie & Co and its colophon are trademarks of Cyre' Marie & Co.

For information about special discounts for bulk purchases, please contact:
hello@cyremarie.com

Manufactured in the United States and distributed globally

ISBN 979-8-3147877-0-0 (Paperback)
ISBN 979-8-9929229-1-2 (Ebook)

Dedication

Mommy
What do you give the woman who not only gave you life but spoke life into you every step of the way? No dream was too big, no idea too wild— you never placed limits on me. Whether I wanted to be an astronaut, a fashion designer, or start a business making purses from scratch, you never doubted me—you just supported me.

You poured into me, sacrificed for me, and lifted me up even when life was heavy on your shoulders. Because of you, I have never been afraid to dream, try, or fail. I stand on the foundation you built, and I am who I am because of you.

I don't say it enough—thank you. I love you endlessly.

Darrell,
My love, my rock—thank you for always being in my corner. You support my dreams, push me when I need it, and inspire me every single day. Through every idea, every late-night brainstorming session, every doubt, and every win—you are right there, believing in me even when I forget to believe in myself. I love you endlessly.

Ocean & October,
Reach for the stars, Kid O's. Your dreams have no boundaries. The world is yours—there's nothing you can't do. Watching you grow reminds me every day that magic exists, and it lives within you both.

Zaniyah
TT's Baby, you did that! Graduating HS with honors—what an accomplishment! TT is so proud of you! You are so smart, so kind, and truly such a beautiful soul. This book is dedicated to you because I know you are about to step into the world and make it yours. Never shrink yourself, never doubt yourself, and never stop reaching for what you want. You are powerful, and I love you so much.

Cyre

And to you, the reader,
I see you. I am proud of you for choosing yourself, for realizing that you
can't pour from an empty cup, and for taking this step toward self-care.
You deserve this journey, and I'm honored to walk alongside you.

—Cyre' Marie

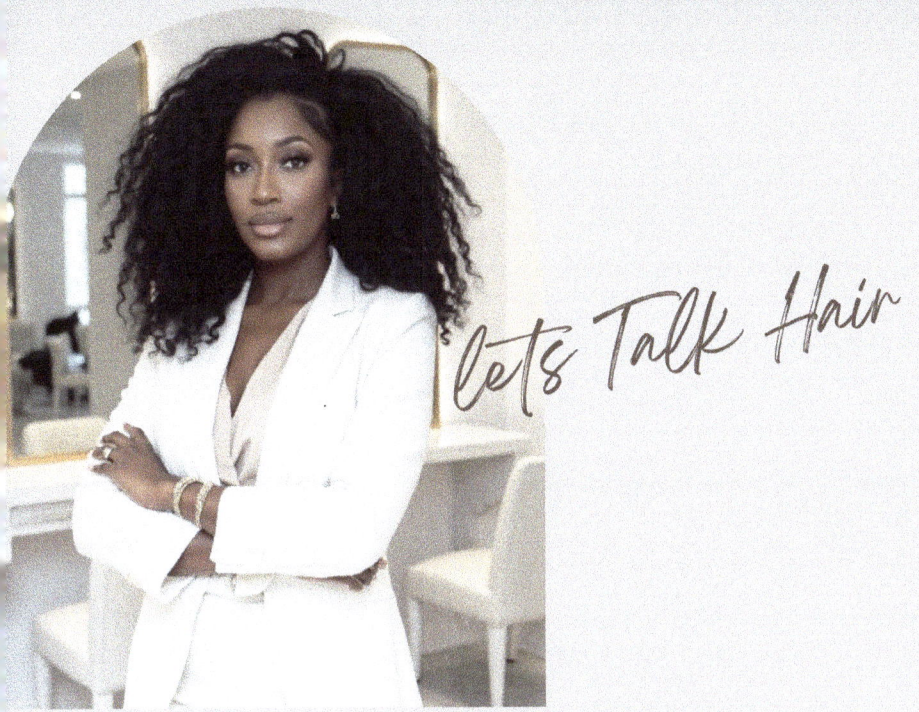

lets Talk Hair

I am Cyre' Marie

your Healthy Hair Bestie— Licensed Cosmetologist of 16 years & honestly, it Always gave Hair Guru. Whether you're flipping through this book for tips or just here for the tea on how to keep your strands thriving, I've got you!

I've styled everyone from your faves on the red carpet to the girl next door, and the mission is always the same: healthy, fabulous hair. As the founder of Hair Therapy, I'm here to give you all the gems—expertise (and a few of my favorite tips and DIY recipes) no gatekeeping— because great hair is a flex and a lifestyle. Let's get into it!

Table of **Contents**

Welcome to Your Hair Therapy Session

Alright, let's clear the air: licensed cosmetologist for 16 years? I know you're trying to do the math—just know I started in this business when I was like 9 (wink wink). What's important is I've been in this game long enough to know what works, what doesn't, and how to help your hair thrive.

Let me say this loud and clear: I am NOT a wig or weave hater. You'll catch me rocking a 30-inch bust-down lace wig one month and boho knotless braids the next. But here's the tea—it's not about what's on top; it's about what's underneath. Your real hair deserves love, too! I'm always checking in with mine like, "Hey girl, you good? Alright, cool—next look incoming!"

Let's be real: salon experiences haven't always been amazing. Maybe you've been burned (literally), left waiting, or feeling overcharged. I get it, and that's why this book exists—to rebuild trust. Trust in stylists, but more importantly, trust in yourself. You're the queen of your hair journey, and I'm just here to hand you the keys.

Inside, you'll find advice for all hair textures, DIY recipes, tips to nourish your hair from the inside out, and a journaling section to track your progress. Quick disclaimer: I'm a licensed cosmetologist, not a doctor. If something feels off-off, call a professional. Self-care means knowing when to tag in backup.

Hair care is a journey—a marathon, not a sprint. Through it all, I'll be your hair expert, your cheerleader, and your hair bestie. But the real magic happens when you commit to showing up for your crown.

Let's do this, babe. Your hair deserves the royal treatment—and trust me, you're in the right place.

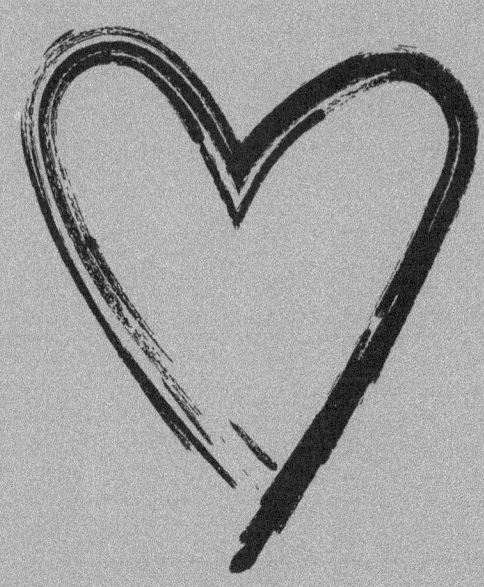

THE PLEDGE
A Love Letter to Our Hair

For far too long, we have been taught to see our hair as a challenge, an inconvenience, or something to "fix." This belief has been ingrained in us not just by society, but by brands, stylists, and sometimes even our own families. It shows up in the way we speak about our hair—calling it "nappy," "unmanageable," or comparing it to a false standard of what "good hair" is supposed to be.

Today, that ends.

Just recently, I had a client sit in my chair and, before I even touched her hair, she sighed and spoke about it with frustration, listing all the reasons she hated it. I have also worked with major beauty brands—some of which claim to serve us, yet behind closed doors, they see our hair as nothing more than a problem to be solved. I have seen marketing teams—ones that do not look like us—script messages that call our hair "nappy" or frame it as something undesirable, as if our natural beauty needs an apology. I experienced this firsthand while working with a brand on a campaign. As I read through the script they provided, I was stopped in my tracks by the opening words: "I hate my hair."

I immediately felt anger and sadness. How could I say that? How could I, someone who has spent years uplifting my clients, encouraging my daughter to love every strand of her natural hair, and embracing the beauty of our hair textures, allow those words to come out of my mouth? No paycheck, no partnership, no marketing campaign is worth denouncing my beauty or the beauty of my people. I refused to say it. I brought my concerns to the company, and though they agreed to remove those words, the damage had already been done.

Their perspective was clear—they saw us as a market, not a people. This moment reinforced something for me: words have power.

The way we speak about our hair shapes the way we treat it. If we constantly call it a burden, we will handle it with frustration. If we call it beautiful, we will nurture it with love. Just like with our skin, nails, and overall self-care, our hair flourishes when we take the time to understand and care for it properly. But before we can even get to that step, we must first change our mindset.

This is why I am including The Hair Pledge. This is not just another page in this book—it is a commitment to speak life into our hair. It is a promise to ourselves to love, respect, and care for our hair with patience and pride.

The Hair Pledge

I pledge to love my hair.
I pledge to be patient with my hair.
I pledge to speak positively about my hair.
I pledge to nourish my hair the way it deserves.
I pledge to embrace my unique texture.
I pledge to let go of old beliefs that tell me my hair is anything less than beautiful.
My hair is not a problem to be fixed. It is a crown to be worn with pride.
Today and every day, I honor my hair.

Signature _____

(Write your name here as a commitment to this pledge.)

Let this be the start of a new relationship with your hair. One filled with love, care, and confidence. Because the way we treat our hair begins with the way we see it—and we will see it for what it is: beautiful.

REMINDER

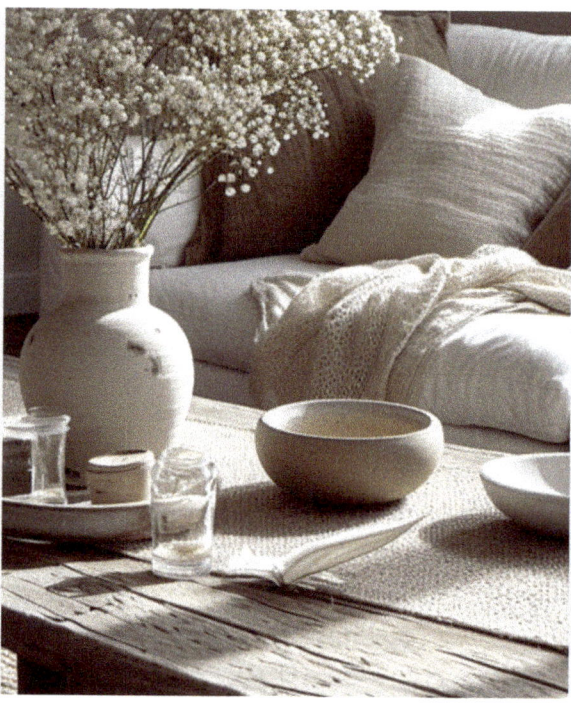

Healthy hair growth takes time—nourish it with care, patience, and love. Trust the process, and your hair will thank you.

Close

1
Chapter

SALON VISITS AND AT-HOME CARE

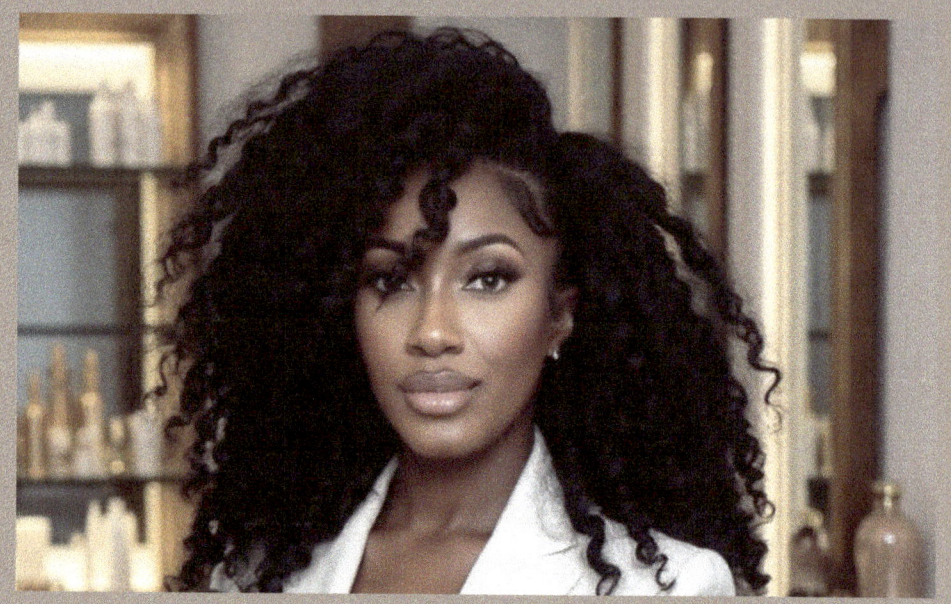

While empowering you to take control of your own hair care is my goal, let's not overlook the value of finding a stylist who truly understands your hair's needs. A great stylist is more than just someone who makes you hair "LOOK good" —they're a partner in your healthy hair journey. Whether it's a trim every 6-8 weeks, managing new growth, or addressing specific concerns like dryness or scalp issues, professional care plays a key role in maintaining your hair's integrity. Using Chemicals, certain services & specialty treatments are sometimes best left to the pros who have the tools and techniques to get the job done right.

That said, the magic really happens in the time between salon visits. A consistent hair care routine tailored to your hair type and needs is crucial. This includes regular moisturizing, protecting your hair at night with a satin or silk scarf, and avoiding excessive heat styling. What you do at home sets the foundation for long-term hair health and helps prolong the benefits of those salon visits.

Understanding Your Hair Alright, let's get real—you can't take care of your hair if you don't actually know your hair. Think of this as a first date with your strands. Is your hair curly, coily, wavy, or rocking its own thing somewhere in between? Knowing your texture is the first step to picking products and styling techniques that actually work. But texture is only part of the story. You also need to figure out what's going on under the hood. Is your hair living its best life, or is it throwing a tantrum because it's dry, brittle, or straight-up damaged? Here's how to figure it out:

- Does your hair stretch without snapping when it's wet? (If it does, she's got elasticity!)

- Does it feel rough, smooth, or like the inside of a Brillo pad? (Be honest—it's just us here.)

Is it shiny and vibrant, or is it giving "I've been through it" vibes? These little tests will tell you what your hair's been up to and what it might need to get back on track. To make it easy, let's break your hair's current mood into four categories:

- Healthy Hair: She's strong, shiny, and unbothered by breakage.m

- Dry Hair: Feels like a cactus, frizzes out at the slightest hint of humidity, and is begging for moisture.

- Brittle Hair: Breaks if you look at it wrong, has split ends for days, and is hard to manage.

- Damaged Hair: This one's in full SOS mode—thanks to heat or chemicals, it's dull, breaking off, and needs some serious TLC.

Is Your Hair in Distress? Let's Fix That.

Let's talk about hair damage—it's like the stages of a bad relationship. First, there's Dry Hair: your hair is feeling neglected and rough, frizzing out like it's throwing a tantrum. This usually happens when your strands are screaming for moisture, thanks to things like sun exposure, harsh shampoos, or just life in general. Then we've got Brittle Hair, where dryness takes a turn for the worse. Now your hair is weak, breaking off when you so much as look at it wrong, dull, and rocking split ends like it's a trend. Finally, there's Damaged Hair, the hair equivalent of rock bottom. This is the result of over-processing with chemicals, frying it with heat tools, or both. It's rough, limp, and snapping like a cheap rubber band.

Now, let's get to the good stuff—how to fix it. First, grab those scissors (or call your stylist!) and commit to regular trims every 6-8 weeks. Split ends? Gone. Next, step away from the flat iron and curling wand. If you must use heat, promise me you'll use a heat protectant spray and the lowest setting possible. Stock your bathroom with hair products that hydrate and repair: think deep conditioning masks, sulfate-free shampoos, and leave-in conditioners. Look for powerhouse ingredients like shea butter, argan oil, and keratin—they're like a spa day for your hair. Feeling extra proactive? Add some hair-friendly vitamins to your routine, like biotin, vitamin E, or omega-3s, to support growth and overall health from the inside out.

The truth is, hair damage doesn't disappear overnight (I wish it did!), but with patience, the right products, and a little TLC, you'll be on your way to shiny, strong, and healthy strands that won't betray you at the first sign of a hairbrush.

2

Chapter

UNDERSTANDING
YOUR HAIR

UNDERSTANDING YOUR HAIR

What's Your Hair Type? Let's Decode It Together

Figuring out your hair type is like finding the right TikTok niche—it's all about knowing what works for you. Hair types are defined by the shape of your hair follicles, which determines your curl pattern, texture, and even how much moisture your hair can hold (a.k.a. porosity). Whether you're rocking Type 1 straight strands, Type 2 waves, Type 3 curls, or Type 4 coils, knowing your type helps you choose the right products and techniques so your hair can thrive.

Now, let's talk curly and coily hair (shoutout to my Type 3s and Type 4s). While these textures are chef's kiss beautiful, they can come with a few challenges—like dryness, shrinkage, and brittleness. Picture this: you've spent an hour detangling, applying your leave-in, and defining every curl, and then BOOM, your hair shrinks like it's dodging a paparazzi camera. Type 4 hair, especially, can be fragile, needing extra TLC to avoid breakage from heat, chemicals, or overhandling.

If this is starting to feel like a science lecture—sorry, not sorry. I promise, this stuff is important! Whether your hair's a springy Type 4 coil like mine or a sleek Type 1, the goal is the same: finding what works for you. Hair care isn't about forcing your strands to behave like someone else's; it's about treating them with the love and patience they deserve. Because when you truly know your hair, you can give it everything it needs to thrive—and trust me, it will thank you for it.

THE FOUR DIFFERENT TYPES OF HAIR TEXTURES

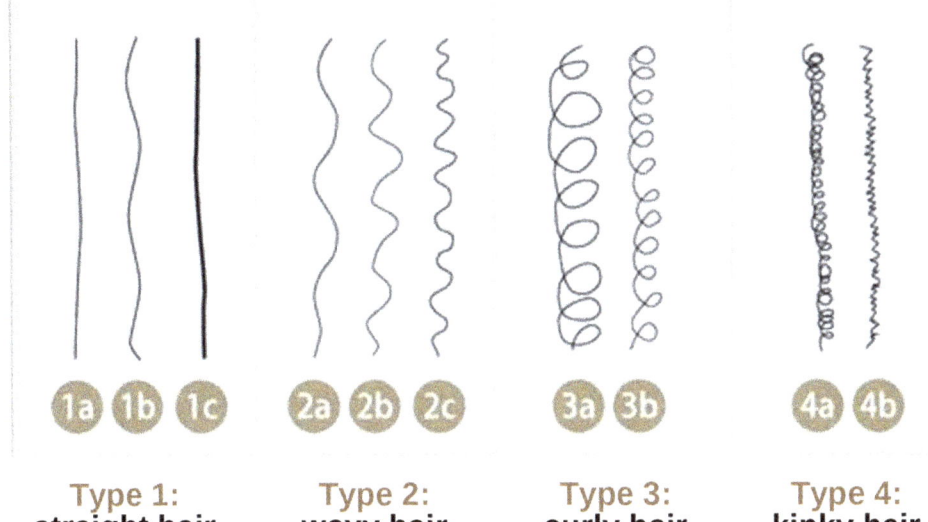

| Type 1: straight hair | Type 2: wavy hair | Type 3: curly hair | Type 4: kinky hair |

HAIR TEXTURE BASICS: WHAT'S YOUR TYPE?

Hair texture is typically classified into four main types:

- Type 1 (straight)
- Type 2 (wavy)
- Type 3 (curly)
- Type 4 (coily/kinky)

Each type has its own unique personality and deserves its own hair care strategy. Let's break it down so you can figure out what works for your strands—no matter where they fall on the texture spectrum!

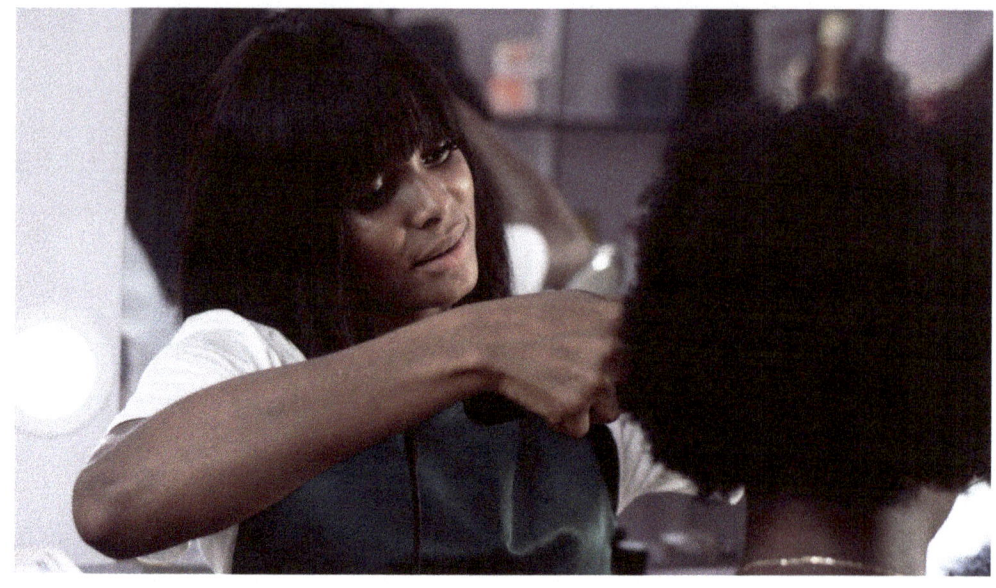

Type 01 **Hair:** Straight

Personality:

Type 1 hair is sleek, straight, and often the envy of anyone who's ever struggled to get a smooth blowout. Natural oils travel easily down the shaft, making it naturally shiny—but sometimes too shiny (hello, greasy roots). Volume can also be a challenge because Type 1 hair tends to lay flat.

Care Tips:

- Use lightweight shampoos and conditioners to avoid buildup.
- Dry shampoo is your best friend for keeping oil at bay between washes.
- Add texture and body with mousses, sprays, or a quick TikTok-inspired blowout hack.

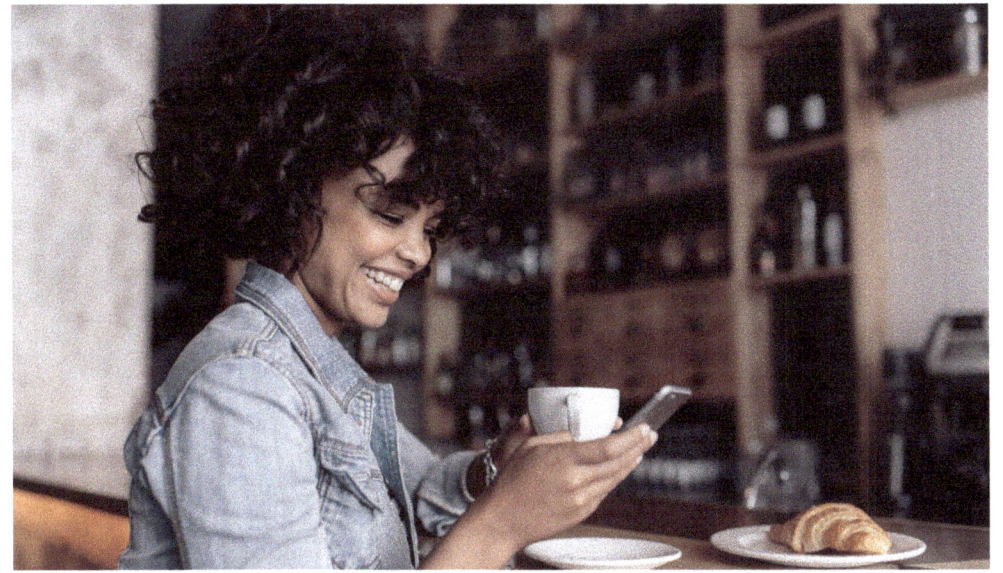

Type 02 Hair: Wavy

Personality:

Type 2 hair is the cool kid that always looks like it just got back from the beach. Its natural waves can range from loose and carefree to more defined S-shaped patterns. While versatile, it's prone to frizz and can lose its wave definition if not cared for properly.

Care Tips:

- Stick to sulfate-free shampoos and conditioners to maintain moisture.
- Use curl-enhancing products like lightweight gels or mousses to define waves.
- Diffuse-dry for that effortless, beachy look—or let it air dry for a softer vibe.

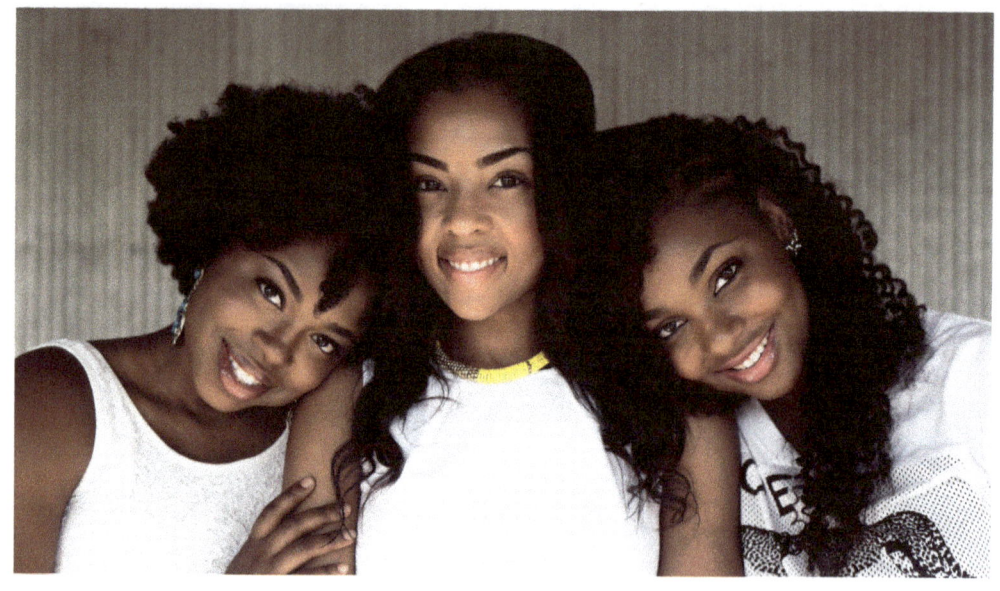

Type 03 **Hair: Curly**

Personality:

Type 3 hair is the life of the party, with curls ranging from playful spirals to tight corkscrews. But like the party guest who shows up with 50 outfit changes, it can be high-maintenance—prone to frizz, dryness, and needing constant hydration.

Care Tips:

- Sulfate-free shampoos are a must to prevent moisture loss.
- Deep condition regularly to keep curls hydrated and bouncy.
- Use curl creams or gels to define your curls while keeping frizz in check.
- Protective styles like twists or braids can help minimize manipulation.

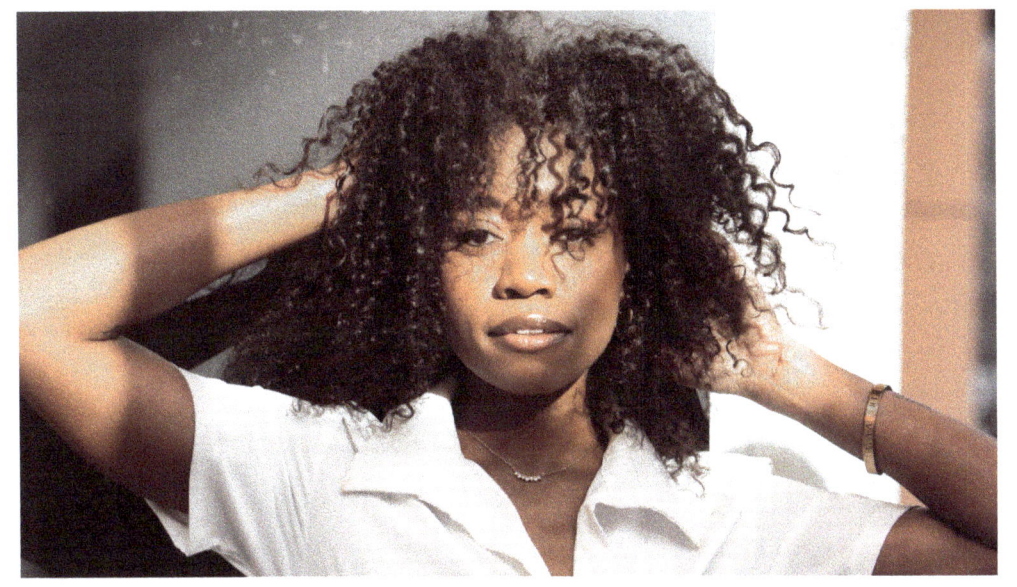

Type 04 Hair: Coily Curly Hair

Personality:

Type 4 hair is the queen of versatility, rocking tight coils, kinks, and gorgeous volume. It's the most delicate of all textures, craving constant hydration and extra TLC. It thrives on routines that prioritize moisture and gentle handling.

Care Tips:

- Co-wash (using conditioner instead of shampoo) to gently cleanse without stripping oils.
- Deep condition regularly to keep coils moisturized and healthy.
- Seal in moisture with thick creams or oils.
- Protective styles like bantu knots, twists, or braids help retain length and reduce breakage.

Hair Textures Continued

No matter your type, learning your hair's unique needs is like figuring out its love language. Whether it's Type 1 sleek or Type 4 coily, your hair deserves a little extra attention and care to help it thrive. So, grab your favorite products, turn on a YouTube tutorial, and let's get those strands looking and feeling their best!

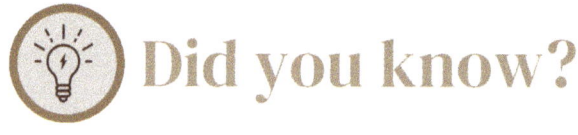 **Did you know?**

A balanced diet rich in vitamins such as biotin, zinc, and iron can significantly impact hair growth and strength.

HAIR GROWTH CYCLE

Your hair's growth cycle is like a well-rehearsed play, with three distinct acts: Anagen, Catagen, and Telogen. Each phase plays a role in the growth, rest, and renewal of your strands. Understanding these stages can help you grasp why your hair grows (or sheds!) the way it does.

THE HAIR GROWTH CYCLE

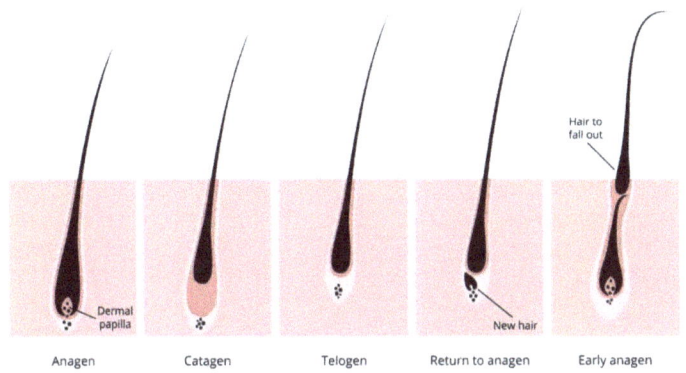

Anagen Catagen Telogen Return to anagen Early anagen

Anagen Phase: The Growth Spurt

This is the star of the hair growth show—the active growth phase. During the anagen phase, cells in the hair root divide like they're on a mission, pushing the hair shaft out of the follicle. For most people, this phase lasts anywhere from 2 to 7 years (lucky genetics can make it even longer). The longer your hair stays in this phase, the longer it can grow.

However, factors like genetics, age, health, and hormones influence how long this phase lasts. For example, someone with a shorter anagen phase might struggle to grow hair beyond a certain length. So if you're eyeing waist-length strands, blame your biology, not your stylist.

Catagen Phase: The Pause Button

The catagen phase is the shortest chapter in the hair growth cycle, lasting just 2 to 3 weeks. This is the transition period where active growth halts, and the hair follicle starts to shrink like it's clocking out for the day. During this phase, the hair separates from its blood supply (aka, the dermal papilla) and gets ready to take a well-deserved rest.

Even though this phase is brief, it's a crucial part of the cycle. Think of it as a reset button, preparing the hair for what's to come.

Telogen Phase: The Pause Button

Finally, we have the telogen phase, the chill-out stage of the hair growth cycle. This resting period lasts about 3 to 4 months, during which the hair strand hangs out in the follicle without growing. At the end of this phase, the hair is shed (totally normal—50 to 100 strands a day, FYI), and the cycle begins anew as a new strand takes its place.

If you notice excessive shedding, it could be a sign of a disruption in the hair growth cycle, often triggered by stress, health concerns, or poor nutrition. But don't panic—there are ways to address this!

Factors Affecting Hair Growth

So, what affects how this whole process plays out? Several factors come into play:
• Genetics: Your DNA determines how long your anagen phase lasts, your hair's maximum growth potential, and its overall health.
• Age: As you age, the cycle shortens, leading to thinner, less dense hair.
• Health and Nutrition: Your hair loves a balanced diet rich in vitamins and minerals. Think biotin, iron, and omega-3s for that extra boost.
• Lifestyle: Chronic stress, lack of sleep, and improper hair care routines can throw your cycle out of whack. (Pro tip: Stress less and sleep more –your hair will thank you!)

Understanding these factors helps you take control of your hair's health. Whether it's adjusting your diet, tweaking your routine, or finding ways to relax, a little effort can make a big difference.

Factors Affecting Hair Growth

The hair growth cycle is a natural rhythm happening behind the scenes 24/7. When you understand how it works and what affects it, you can take steps to support your hair's health and growth. So whether you're in the growth spurt, the pause button, or the shedding phase, know that your hair is doing its thing–and you can help it along the way!

HAIR POROSITY 101:

Is Your Hair Playing Hard to Get or Too Easy?

Alright, sis, let's talk porosity—because knowing your hair's porosity level is like knowing if it's a low-maintenance boo or if it needs constant attention (we've all been there). Understanding porosity will help you pick the right products, avoid product buildup disasters, and keep your hair thriving like it just walked out of a salon (without breaking the bank).

So, what exactly is hair porosity? In short, it's how well your hair can absorb and retain moisture. Think of it like dating—some hair types play hard to get (low porosity), while others fall in love too quickly (high porosity). And then there's the perfect match in between (normal porosity).

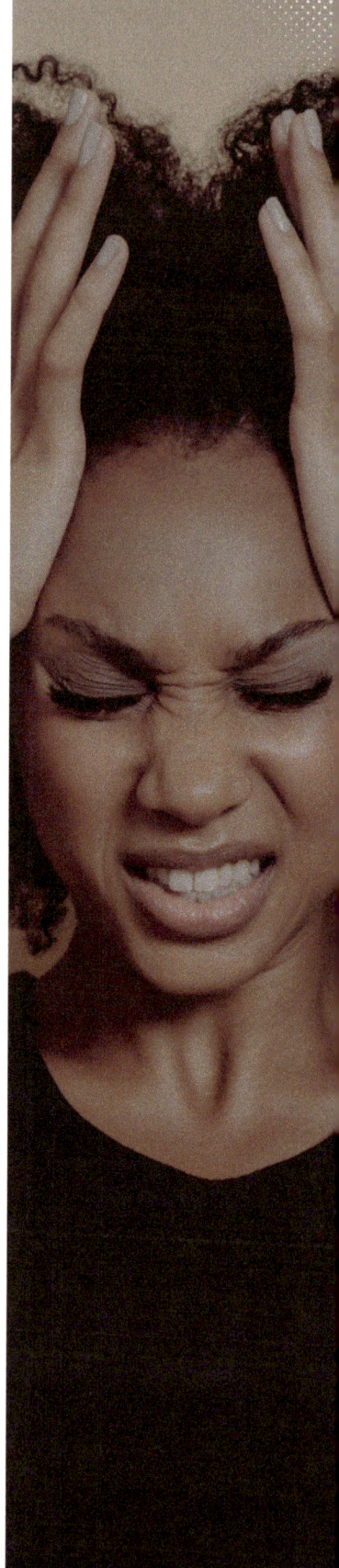

Low Porosity: The Hard-to-Get Diva

If your hair is low porosity, it's basically got trust issues. It resists moisture like it's dodging an ex's text messages. Your cuticles (the outer layer of your hair) are tight and closed off, making it tough for water and products to penetrate.

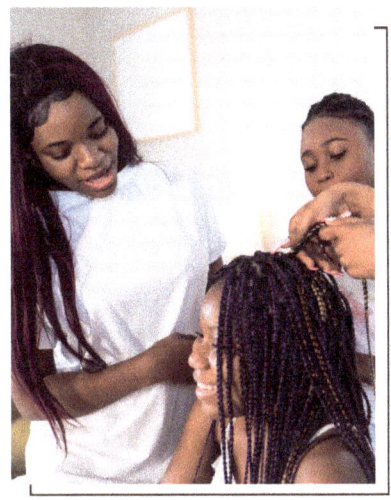

How to Tell If You Have Low Porosity Hair:

- Water beads up and sits on top of your strands instead of soaking in.

- Products just sit there, making you look like you overdid it on the leave-in.

- Your hair takes forever (and I mean forever) to fully dry.

- Heat styling? It's a struggle—your hair doesn't want to play nice.

> **The Float Test:** Fill a glass with water and drop a clean, shed hair into it. If it floats like it's chilling on vacation, congratulations—you've got low porosity hair.

DISCLAIMER:
Read This Before You DIY!

Listen, I'm here to empower you to take control of your hair journey—but I've got to say it: I'm not a doctor, dermatologist, or miracle worker (although I do know my way around a good hair mask!). Everything in this book is based on my personal experience, research, and passion for healthy hair. But here's the deal:

➤ Patch Test Everything! Just because it works for me (and thousands of others) doesn't mean it's a perfect match for you. Always test a small area before going all in.

➤ Consult the Pros. If you have allergies, medical conditions, or serious hair/scalp concerns, it's always best to check with a licensed professional before trying anything new.

➤ Results May Vary. Hair is unique—what works wonders for one person might not be the magic potion for another. Stay consistent and listen to your hair.

Basically, I'm here to guide and inspire, but I can't be held responsible for any unexpected hair adventures (good or bad). So, take what works for you, have fun experimenting, and always put your hair's health first!

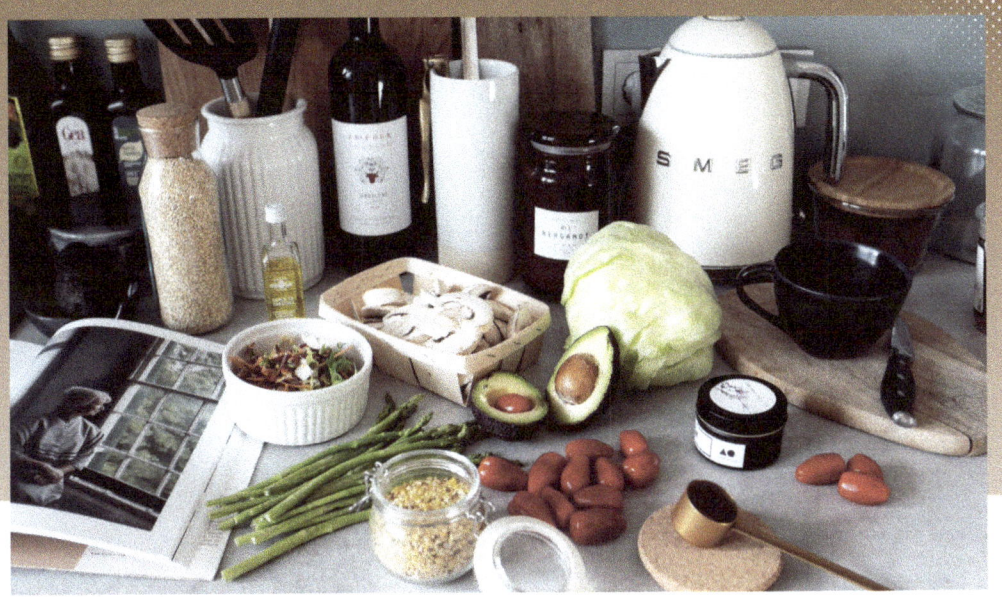

DIY RECIPE FOR LOW POROSITY HAIR:

Hydration Boost Steam Mask

- 1/2 cup aloe vera gel (because moisture is life)1 tbsp light coconut oil (penetrates deeper)
- 1 tbsp honey (nature's humectant)
- 1 tbsp apple cider vinegar (to help open the cuticle)

Directions:

Mix all ingredients, apply to damp hair, and cover with a plastic cap. Sit under a steamer or use a warm towel for 20 minutes. Your hair will thank you later.

High Porosity: The Thirsty Babe

Now, if your hair is high porosity, it's basically the friend who spills all their secrets too fast. It soaks up moisture like crazy–but the problem? It lets it go just as fast. Your cuticles are wide open like an "enter at your own risk" sign, which means your hair is prone to frizz, dryness, and breakage.

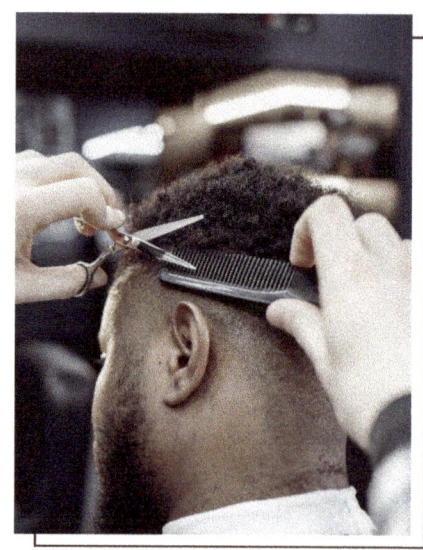

How to Tell If You Have High Porosity Hair:

- Your hair drinks up products like a smoothie, but an hour later? Bone dry.

- It frizzes up at the slightest hint of humidity (thanks, weather).

- Your strands snap off easily like they're going through something.

- It air-dries way too quickly.

> **The Spray Test:** Lightly mist your hair with water. If it absorbs almost instantly, you've got high porosity hair.

DIY RECIPE FOR HIGH POROSITY HAIR:

Moisture Lock Deep Conditioner

- 1/2 ripe avocado (healthy fats for strength)
- 2 tbsp shea butter (hello, moisture retention!)
- 1 tbsp castor oil (keeps moisture locked in)
- 1 tbsp honey (because we stay sweet)

Directions:

Blend all ingredients into a creamy mixture, apply generously to damp hair, and let it marinate under a plastic cap for 30 minutes before rinsing. Follow up with a cool rinse to help seal the cuticles.

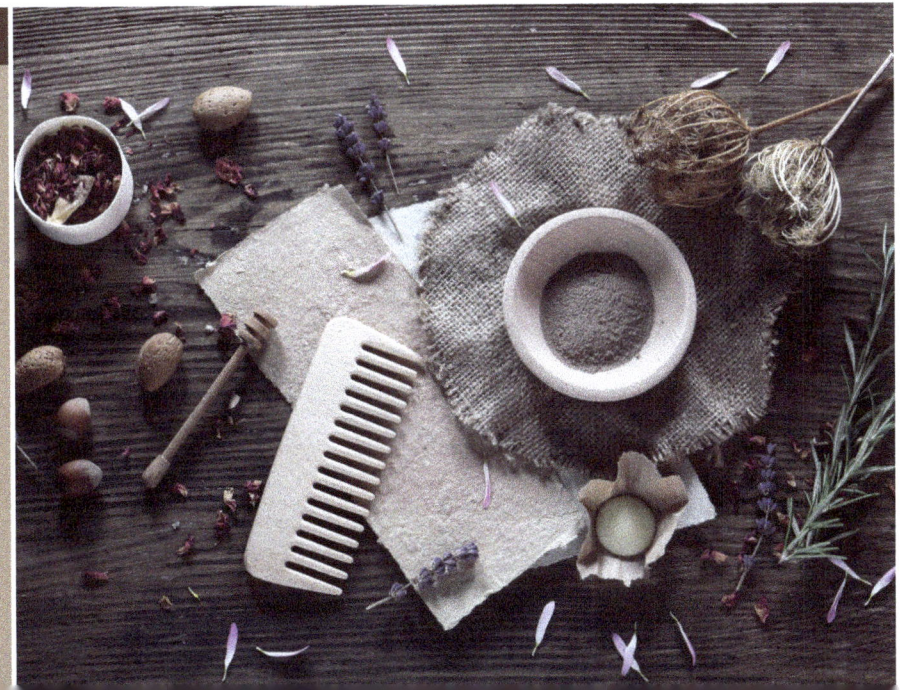

NORMAL POROSITY:
THE EASYGOING QUEEN

If you've got normal porosity, count your blessings, sis! Your hair knows how to take in moisture and hold onto it like a healthy relationship. It's not too picky with products and generally behaves itself.

▶ **How to Tell If You Have Normal Porosity Hair:**

- Your hair absorbs moisture and holds onto it without much drama.

- It air-dries in a reasonable amount of time—neither too fast nor too slow.

- Styles actually last without looking like a frizzy mess halfway through the day.

- It's got that healthy bounce and shine.

> **The Slip 'N Slide Test:** When you apply product, your hair absorbs it evenly without getting too greasy or dry. If it feels balanced, you're good to go.

> Now that you know what you're working with, let's talk about how to keep your hair living its best life:

Low Porosity Queens:

- Use heat (steam caps, warm water) to open those cuticles.
- Lightweight oils are your BFF—think argan or grapeseed oil.
- Avoid product buildup by using clarifying shampoos.

High Porosity Babes:

- Always seal with heavier oils and butters (shea, castor oil).
- Use protein treatments to strengthen your strands.
- Rinse with cool water to close those cuticles after conditioning.

Normal Porosity Girls:

- Maintain balance—don't overdo it with too much protein or moisture.
- Stick to a solid routine and enjoy the best of both worlds.
- Protective styles can help retain your hair's natural moisture levels.

Final Thoughts

Porosity isn't just a buzzword—it's the key to unlocking your hair's full potential. Whether your hair is high-maintenance or chill, understanding porosity helps you give it exactly what it needs. And remember, no matter your hair type, the goal is always healthy, thriving hair that's as fabulous as you are.

3

Chapter

WEATHERING YOUR HAIR

Listen, love—your hair is just like your wardrobe. You wouldn't rock a fur coat in the middle of summer, right? Well, your hair needs the same seasonal adjustment. Whether you're battling the humid streets of Atlanta, the dry desert air of Phoenix, or the chilly winds of New York, your hair feels every shift in the atmosphere.

So, let's get into it—how different climates and seasons play with your strands and what you can do to stay ahead of Mother Nature's antics. Because trust me, she's not always on our side.

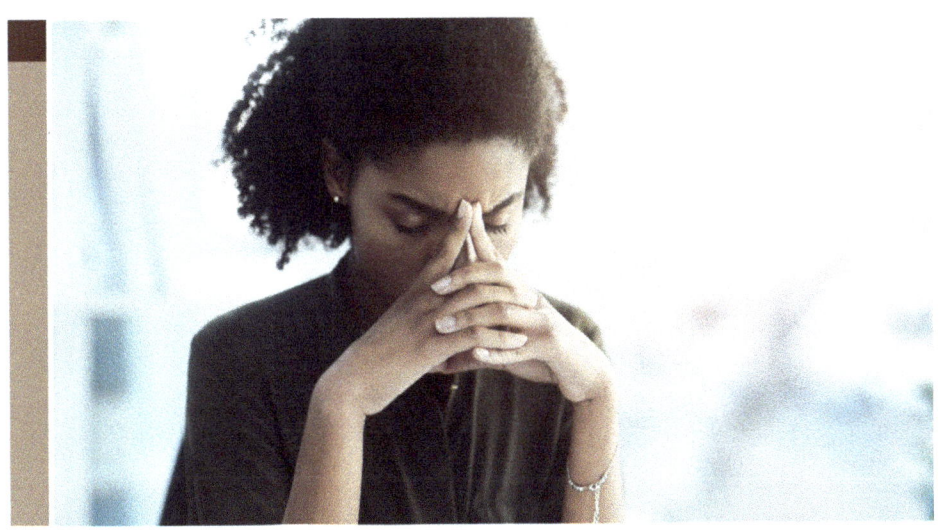

HOT & HUMID WEATHER: WHEN YOUR HAIR FEELS LIKE IT'S MELTING

Humidity—aka the arch-nemesis of a good silk press. You step outside looking like a goddess, and five minutes later, poof! Your hair has its own weather system. Humid climates (think Florida, Louisiana, or any tropical vacation spot) are all about excess moisture in the air, which your hair loves to drink up—sometimes too much.

▶ **How Humidity Affects Your Hair:**

- High porosity hair = instant frizz. Your strands soak up water like a sponge, expanding in all the wrong ways.
- Low porosity hair = weighed-down and limp. Moisture sits on top, making your hair feel greasy.
- Your sleek styles? Gone faster than your paycheck on payday.

▶ **Humidity Survival Kit:**

- Anti-humidity products are a MUST. Look for serums with silicones to block moisture from sneaking in.
- Lightweight leave-ins. Heavy products will just attract more moisture—stick to light creams or sprays.
- Protective styles to the rescue. Braids, buns, and twists keep the frizz at bay and your style intact.

▶ **DIY Humidity Shield Spray:**

- 1 cup rose water (because we're fancy like that)
- 1 tbsp argan oil (lightweight and fights frizz)
- 5 drops lavender oil (to keep your scalp calm)
- Spritz before styling and thank me later.

Dry & Cold Weather: The Silent Hair Snatcher

Winter weather is like that toxic ex—dry, cold, and constantly trying to suck the life out of you. If you're living in colder climates (looking at you, Chicago and NYC), you know that winter doesn't just hit your skin; it hits your hair too. The air lacks moisture, your scalp gets dry and flaky, and your ends? Brittle city.

How Cold Weather Affects Your Hair:

- Your hair becomes drier than your DMs on a Sunday morning.
- Breakage is at an all-time high thanks to dry air and friction from scarves and sweaters.
- Wash day takes longer because your hair needs ALL the moisture it can get.

Cold Weather Survival Kit:

- Deep conditioning is non-negotiable. Weekly moisture masks keep your hair soft and hydrated.
- Switch to heavier butters and oils. Shea butter, castor oil, and olive oil help lock in moisture for the long haul.
- Silk-lined hats, please. Wool hats might be cute, but they're low-key damaging your hair.

DIY Winter Rescue Hair Mask:

- 1 ripe banana (hydration queen)
- 2 tbsp shea butter (because winter is ruthless)
- 1 tbsp honey (natural humectant to draw in moisture)
- Blend it up, apply to damp hair, and let it sit for 30 minutes before rinsing.

HOT & DRY WEATHER:
THE SNEAKY DEHYDRATOR

If you're living in dry climates like Phoenix or Las Vegas, girl, your hair is probably screaming for hydration. Dry heat acts like a moisture thief, leaving your strands brittle and lifeless. And don't even think about skipping wash day—your scalp will have thoughts.

How Dry Climates Affect Your Hair:

- Your hair feels rough, stiff, and lifeless (aka desert vibes).
- Your scalp gets flaky, and product buildup happens faster.
- Lightweight oils won't cut it—you need the heavy hitters.

Dry Climate Survival Kit:

- Hydration is key. Use water-based leave-ins daily to keep your strands quenched.
- Say no to alcohol-heavy products. They'll dry your hair out even faster.
- Scalp care is a priority. Oil massages with tea tree or peppermint keep flakes at bay.

DIY Moisture Lock Hair Spray:

- 1 cup aloe vera juice (super hydrating)
- 1 tbsp glycerin (pulls moisture into your hair)
- 1 tbsp coconut oil (to seal it all in)
- Spritz daily, and your hair will be living its best life.

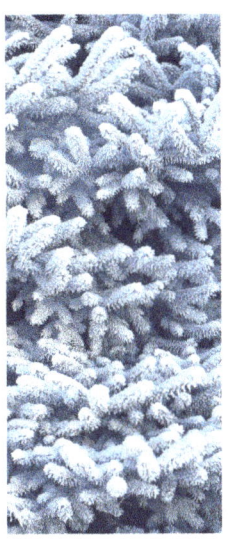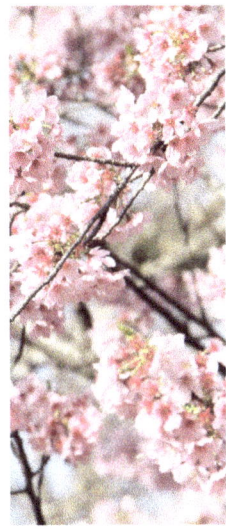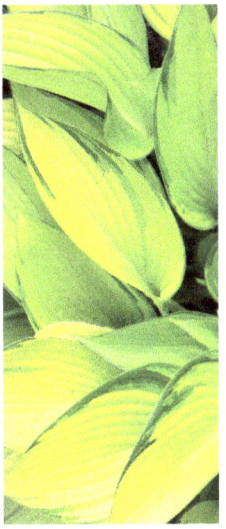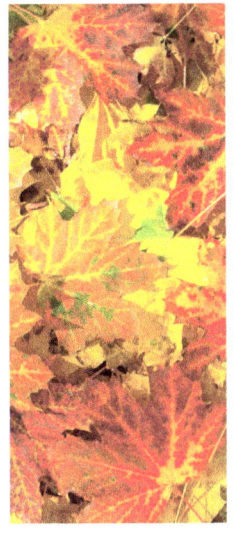

SEASONAL HAIR CARE:

How to Adjust with the Seasons

Think of your hair routine like your skincare routine—what works in the summer won't cut it in the winter. Here's how to switch things up when the seasons change:

Spring:

- Time to repair winter damage with deep conditioning treatments.
- Start incorporating lightweight oils like jojoba to prep for warmer weather.
- Protective styles like braids or buns are great to transition into the summer.

Summer:

- Hydration overload! Leave-in conditioners and anti-humidity sprays are your BFFs.
- Protective styles like twists and updos keep your hair safe from heat and sweat.
- Don't forget scalp protection—sunscreen isn't just for your skin!

Fall:

- Start introducing thicker creams to combat cooler temps.
- Trim those ends to get rid of any summer damage.
- Invest in a silk scarf to protect your hair from windy days.

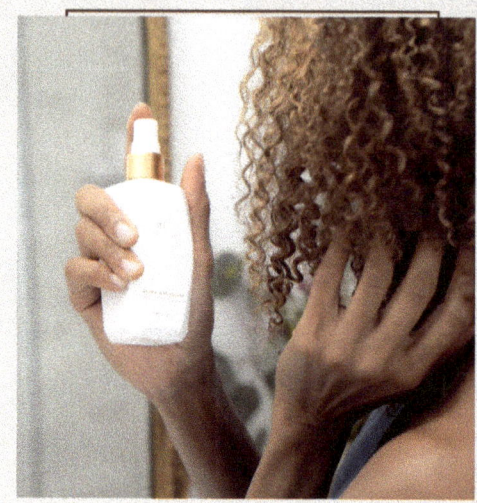

Winter:

- Deep conditioning and heavy butters are your besties.
- Protective styles like wigs and weaves can help protect against breakage.
- Hot oil treatments help combat a dry scalp.

Listen , your hair is in a lifelong relationship with the weather, whether you like it or not. The key to thriving is adapting—just like you swap out your wardrobe, your hair care needs a seasonal refresh too. Stay ahead of the game with the right products, DIY treatments, and protective styles, and your crown will stay flawless no matter the forecast.

So, whether it's hot, cold, humid, or dry—your hair's got this. And with a little TLC, you'll be looking and feeling like the queen you are, year-round.

4

Chapter

CARING FOR
YOUR HAIR

Your Hair Deserves a Little TLC

Hey, gorgeous—let's talk about keeping your hair happy, hydrated, and thriving. Whether your hair is straight, wavy, curly, or coily, these basics will have you flipping it like you're in a shampoo commercial (minus the drama).

Cleanse Like a Boss
First rule: treat your hair gently. Grab a sulfate-free shampoo—because who needs their natural oils snatched? Massage your scalp with your fingertips (think spa vibes, not scrubbing a dirty pan) to remove buildup and boost blood flow. Oh, and skip the hot water. It's not your friend. Lukewarm is the vibe for keeping moisture locked in. Not feeling a full wash? Co-wash with conditioner and keep it moving.

Moisturize & Seal the Deal
Hydration is everything, babe. After washing, hit your hair with a water-based leave-in conditioner to quench its thirst. Then, lock it in with your favorite oil or butter. And don't forget the ends— they're like the elders of your hair, wise but a little fragile. Show them some extra love.

Quick Hair Hacks:
• Listen to your hair: If it's dry or cranky, adjust your routine.
• Be consistent: A little effort every day beats a once-in-a-while deep dive.
• Gentle is the goal: Handle your strands like they're fine silk.

See? Healthy hair doesn't have to be complicated. Just a little love and a good routine, and your strands will be living their best life. Ready to make it happen? Let's go!

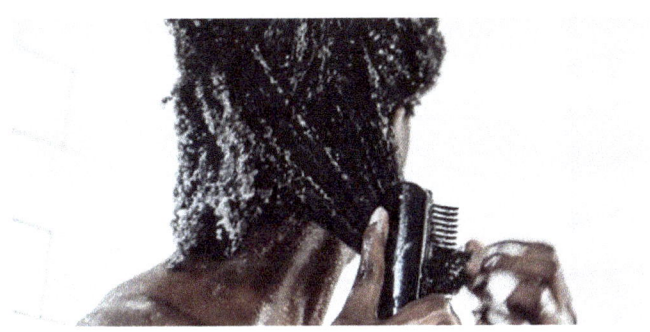

Protective Styles

Let's talk about protective styling—a.k.a. your hair's best friend when it's time to grow, shine, and stay damage-free. Styles like braids, twists, buns, and updos are perfect for giving your hair a break from the daily grind. But let's clear up one thing real quick: that saying "beauty is pain?" Yeah, it's a bold-faced lie. If it's tight enough to make you wince, it's tight enough to cause real damage.

Here's the deal:

Speak up

If your stylist is pulling tighter than a pair of jeans after Thanksgiving dinner, don't stay silent. Let them know—it's your scalp, not theirs!

Post-Style Pain?

Take it out! No temporary look is worth permanent damage. Got it? Good.

While your hair's tucked away in its fabulous protective style, remember to keep it moisturized. Dry hair in braids? That's like leaving your plants in the sun with no water—tragic. Grab your favorite leave-in conditioner or a light oil to keep your strands and scalp happy.

The Break Rules

Protective styles aren't a forever thing (even if you're loving your braids). Give your hair and scalp some breathing room between styles. Overdoing it can lead to breakage, thinning, and all kinds of drama you don't want.

Treatmenths that mean Business

Now, protective styling isn't the whole story. You've got to put in some work to keep your hair thriving. Here's the scoop:

Weekly TLC

Deep condition like your life (or at least your hair's life) depends on it. Look for treatments with hydrating ingredients like honey, aloe vera, and shea butter. These will leave your strands softer than your favorite cashmere sweater.

Monthly Power Moves

Heat and chemicals can do a number on your hair, so bring in the big guns: protein treatments. These strengthen your hair shaft and repair damage. But don't overdo it—too much protein can leave your hair feeling stiff and brittle, and nobody wants that.

Quick Tip: Balance is key! Alternate between moisture and protein treatments to keep your hair strong, soft, and thriving.

So, whether you're rocking a sleek bun or a fresh set of twists, remember: protective styles should protect—not punish. Treat your hair with love, speak up when it's too tight, and keep that scalp hydrated. Your crown deserves the best!

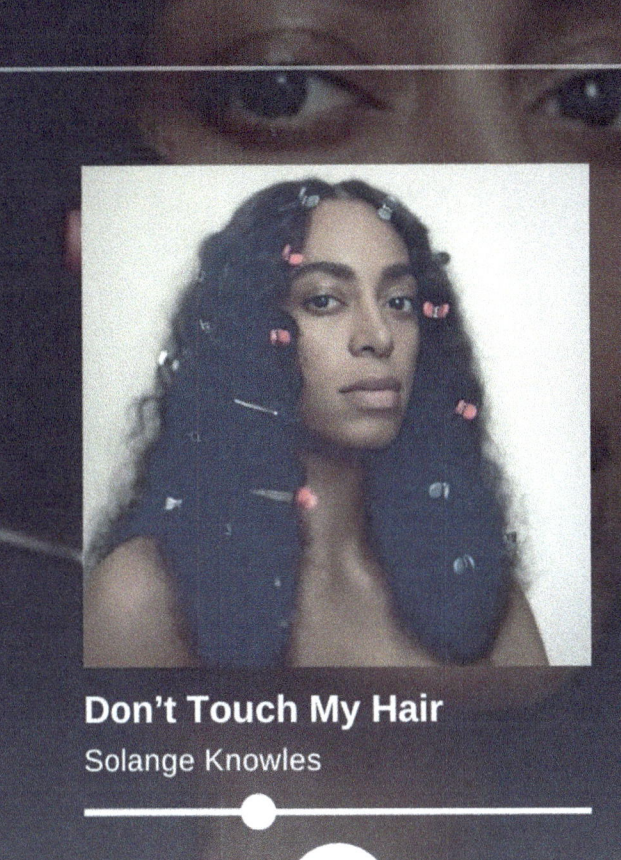

Don't Touch My Hair

Solange Knowles

START

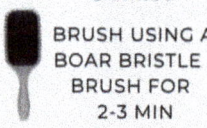

BRUSH USING A
BOAR BRISTLE
BRUSH FOR
2-3 MIN

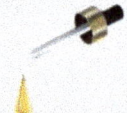

ROSEMARY OIL ON
SCALP

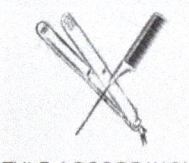

STYLE ACCORDINGLY

MONTHLY
HAIRCARE
ROUTINE

CASTOR OIL
MID LENTH AND
ENDS

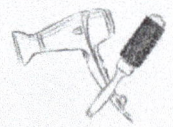

Air Dry or Blow Dry

WAIT 1 - 2 HOURS...

HEAT PROTECTION
SERUM

LEAVE IN
CONDITIONER

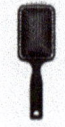

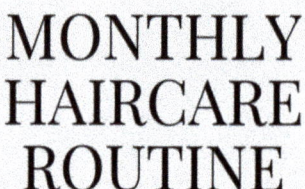

CLARIFYING SHAMPOO
(SKIP CONDITIONER)

MASK

BRUSH

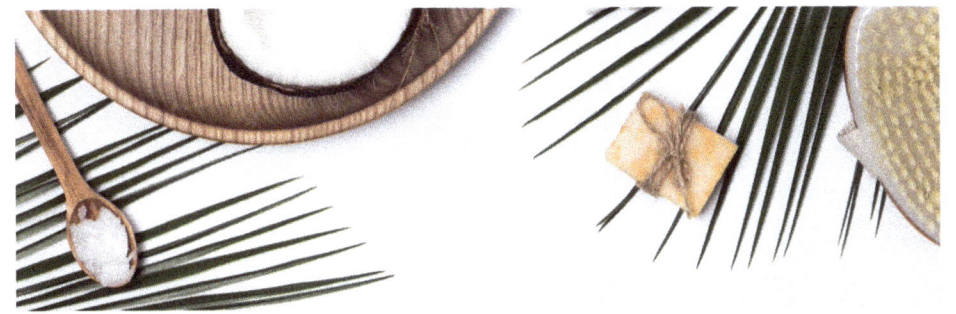

Scalp Massages: Your New Favorite Hobby

Girl, let me put you on game: scalp massages are everything. Not only do they feel amazing, but they're also like a VIP pass for your hair follicles. When you massage your scalp, you're boosting blood flow, which means your roots get all the good nutrients they need to grow and thrive. Think of it as a mini workout for your scalp—except it's totally relaxing and zero sweat involved.

Here's how to do it: grab your fingertips (or a scalp massager if you're feeling fancy) and work that magic daily or a few times a week. Want to level up? Add a few drops of rosemary, peppermint, or lavender oil. Not only do they wake your scalp up in the best way, but the smell? Chef's kiss. Bonus: it's basically aromatherapy for your stress levels, and less stress = happier hair.

Protecting Your Hair at Night: The Real Glow-Up

Sis, your hair deserves beauty sleep, too! That cotton pillowcase you've been sleeping on? It's playing you. Cotton sucks the moisture right out of your hair and leaves it vulnerable to breakage. Switch it up with a satin or silk scarf, bonnet, or pillowcase—it's like wrapping your hair in luxury every night.

And let's talk about heat and chemicals for a second. I get it, you love a sleek press or popping curls, but doing the most every day will have your hair looking stressed and tired. Instead, try air-drying or gentle heat styling, and give those strands a break with low-maintenance styles. Protect your hair like it's the crown it is—because let's be real, it is.

So, are you ready to massage, silk it up, and keep it cute without the drama? Because healthy, strong hair is the real goal, and you've got this. Now go give your scalp some love and tuck that crown in for the night.

What do you think? Does this feel more aligned with your book's vibe? Let me know if we need to tweak it further!

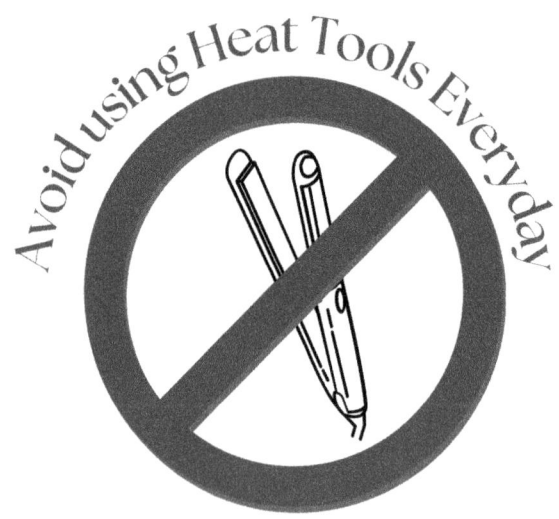

This section is all about understanding your hair, learning how to care for it with love and intention, and discovering practical solutions to support regrowth. Whether you're exploring natural remedies or simply looking for ways to protect your scalp and maintain confidence, I've got you covered.

☐ ## Use Harsh Chemicals

Skip treatments that contain sulfates, parabens, and harsh dyes, which can further irritate the scalp.

☐ ## Skip Moisturizing

Dryness can weaken strands and slow regrowth, so make hydration a priority.

☐ ## Stress Too Much

Easier said than done, but stress management plays a huge role in hair health. Deep breathing, self-care, and mindfulness can make a big difference.

5

Chapter

NATURAL REMEDIES

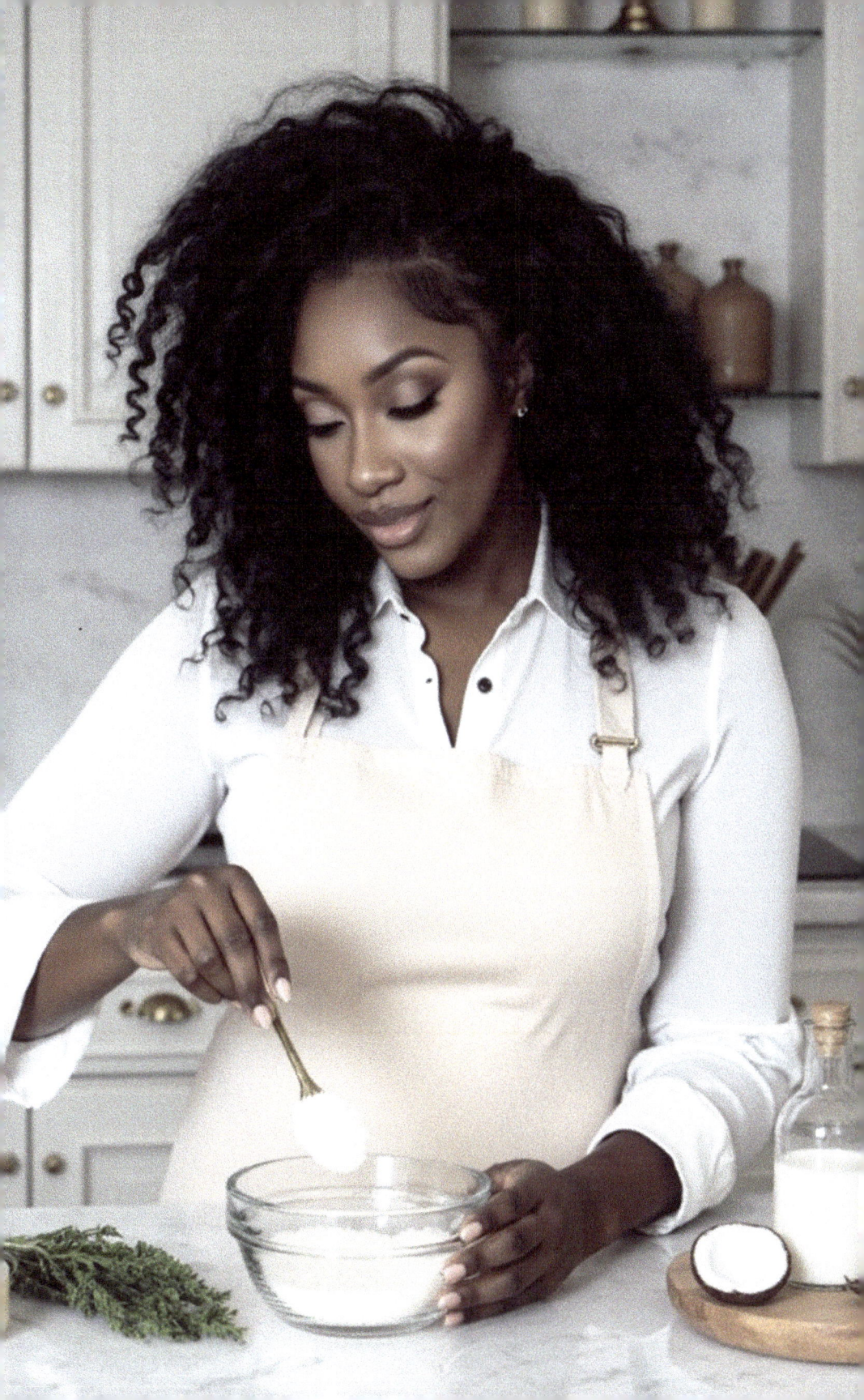

Natural Remedies: Your Hair's New Besties

Listen, sometimes your hair just wants a little love straight from Mother Nature. No chemicals, no drama —just pure, simple magic. Here are two of my favorite go-tos:

Aloe Vera: Your Hair's Hydration BFF

Aloe vera isn't just a sunburn fixer—it's the Beyoncé of natural hair care. Scoop the gel from the leaf, slap it on your scalp and strands, and let it do its thing for 30 minutes. Rinse with lukewarm water (because hot water is not your friend). You'll be left with hydrated, dandruff-free, shiny hair that's basically screaming, "Look at me!"

Hibiscus: The Glow-Up Flower

Hibiscus is like a personal trainer for your hair—full of vitamins and amino acids to keep your strands strong and growing. Blend the petals into a paste with yogurt or coconut oil, pop it on for an hour, and rinse. Boom! Hair so shiny you'll want to twirl it like you're in a hair commercial.

Natural remedies: easy, effective, and a little luxurious. Try these and thank me later—we're in this hair care thing together!

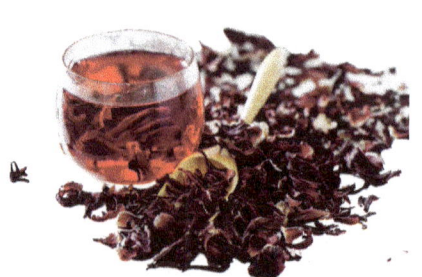

Hair Oils for Scalp Stimulation

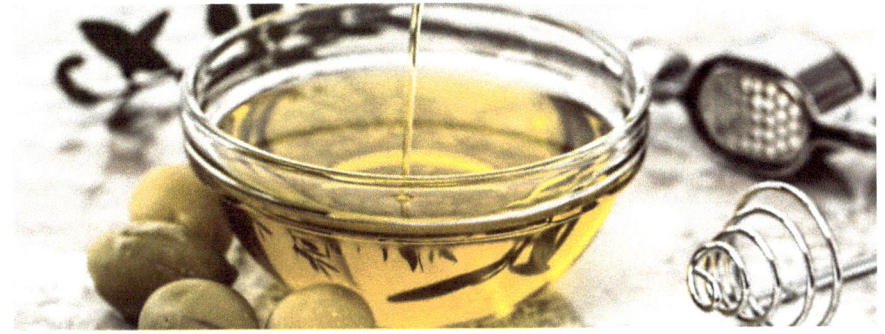

Let's spice up your hair care routine with a couple of heavy hitters: rosemary and peppermint essential oils. These little bottles of magic aren't just good for making your bathroom smell like a spa—they're also hair growth boosters you'll want in your lineup.

Rosemary Oil: The Overachiever

Rosemary oil is like that friend who's good at everything. It improves blood flow to the scalp (hello, growth!), fights dandruff, and even helps keep premature grays at bay. Mix a few drops with a carrier oil like coconut or jojoba, massage it into your scalp, and let it sit for at least 30 minutes. Then wash it out and wait for your scalp to throw you a thank-you party.

Peppermint Oil: The Cool Kid

Peppermint oil brings the vibes and the results. Its cooling effect wakes your scalp up (literally) and gets the blood flowing, which is great for growth. Plus, it's got antimicrobial powers to keep your scalp healthy. Mix a few drops with a carrier oil, rub it in, or sneak some into your shampoo for an extra zing.

Hair Oils for Scalp Stimulation

The Results?
Healthier, stronger hair and a scalp that feels like it's living its best life. Use these oils regularly, and your hair might just start giving shampoo commercial energy. You're welcome.

Does this hit the mark for you? Let me know if you'd like me to tweak anything!

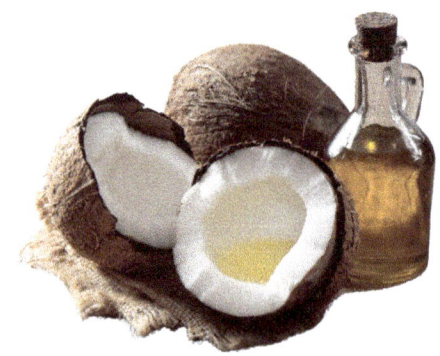

Homemade Hair Masks and Rinses

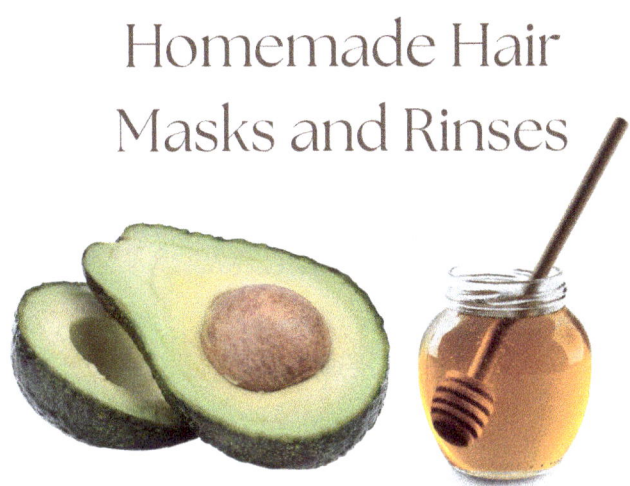

Look, I'm all for a good salon session (obviously, I am the salon), but between appointments, your hair deserves some extra love. These quick DIY treatments are like a love letter to your strands–easy, effective, and totally worth the hype.

Avocado & Honey Mask: Your Hair's Happy Meal

Avocado isn't just for guac, and honey? Not just for tea. Together, they're the Beyoncé and Jay-Z of hair masks: a power couple.

• Mash a ripe avocado (no snacking!) and mix it with two tablespoons of honey.

• Smear that goodness all over your hair and scalp like you're painting a masterpiece.

• Let it marinate for 30 minutes, then rinse. Your hair will be softer, shinier, and more hydrated than a celeb on a green juice cleanse.

Eggs and Castor Oil: The Dynamic Duo Your Hair Will Thank You For

Alright, let's crack (pun intended) into two hair care legends: eggs and castor oil. They're like your hair's personal trainers—building strength, boosting growth, and giving you the main character energy you deserve.

Egg & Olive Oil Mask: A Protein Shake for Your Hair

Eggs aren't just breakfast material—they're packed with protein and biotin, a.k.a. the secret sauce for strong, shiny hair. Add olive oil to the mix, and you've got a moisture-packed dream team.

Here's how to whip it up:
 • Beat two eggs (don't be shy, whisk like a pro) and mix in two tablespoons of olive oil.

 • Slather this magic potion onto your hair and pop on a shower cap—you'll look fabulous, trust me.

 • Let it work its wonders for 20-30 minutes, then rinse with cool water (unless you're into scrambled hair). Follow with a mild shampoo.

The result? Hair so strong and shiny, people might start asking what salon you go to. Just smile and say, "Oh, this? It's homemade."

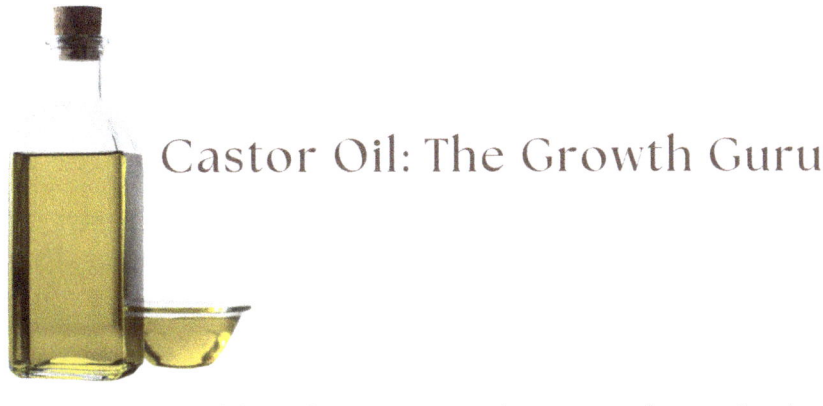

Castor Oil: The Growth Guru

Castor oil is like that overachieving friend who does everything. It's packed with ricinoleic acid and omega-6 fatty acids that stimulate blood flow to your scalp, making your hair thicker, stronger, and ready to slay.
Here's how to use it:

- Warm a small amount (just enough to feel cozy, not lava-hot).

- Massage it into your scalp like you're giving yourself the spa treatment you deserve.

- Leave it overnight (if you can stand the greasiness

-
  shower caps are lifesavers) and rinse it out the next morning with a gentle shampoo.

For an extra boost, mix castor oil with coconut or almond oil. Regular use will have your hair thanking you with volume, strength, and that "just-left-the-salon" vibe.
See? Easy, effective, and totally doable. Now go show your hair some love-it's about to look

Tea Tree Oil: Your Scalp's Ride-or-Die
Scalp Health and Dandruff Prevention

Listen, tea tree oil is like that friend who doesn't just tell you your wig is slipping but helps you fix it in the bathroom. This oil is here to save your scalp, unclog those follicles, and fight dandruff like it owes you money.

Here's the tea mix a few drops of tea tree oil with a carrier oil (because undiluted tea tree is spicy, and we're not trying to burn our scalp off). Massage it in like you're working out all the drama from last week, then let it marinate for 20-30 minutes. Wash it out and voilà, your scalp is feeling fresh and bougie. Pro tip: add a few drops to your shampoo if you're too busy to do the whole oil massage thing every week. Keep at it, and soon you'll be saying, "Dandruff? Never met her."

Lavender Oil: A Chill Pill for Your Scalp

Lavender oil isn't just for making your bedroom smell like a spa–it's here to give your scalp the VIP treatment too. Stress can mess with your edges, sis, but lavender oil is like a deep breath for your hairline. It boosts circulation, helps your hair grow, and smells so good you'll feel like you're on vacation.

Mix a few drops with a carrier oil, and rub it in before bed. Think of it as a scalp massage and aromatherapy in one–who needs a therapist when you've got lavender? Bonus: it might even help you sleep better, which we both know is the real fountain of youth. Stick with it, and soon your hair will be thriving like it just got back from a wellness retreat.

6

Chapter

HAIR CARE ROUTINE

Hair Care Routine

Selecting the right products and treatments is crucial for a successful hair care plan. Choose shampoos, conditioners, and styling products that cater to your hair type and address your specific concerns. For instance, if you have dry hair, opt for moisturizing and hydrating products. For damaged hair, look for strengthening and reparative treatments. Incorporate natural remedies and DIY treatments, such as aloe vera for moisturizing or protein treatments for strengthening, into your routine. Regularly deep condition and use leave-in conditioners to maintain moisture levels and protect your hair from environmental damage.

create a weekly hair care routine, below is an example of a weekly hair care routine.

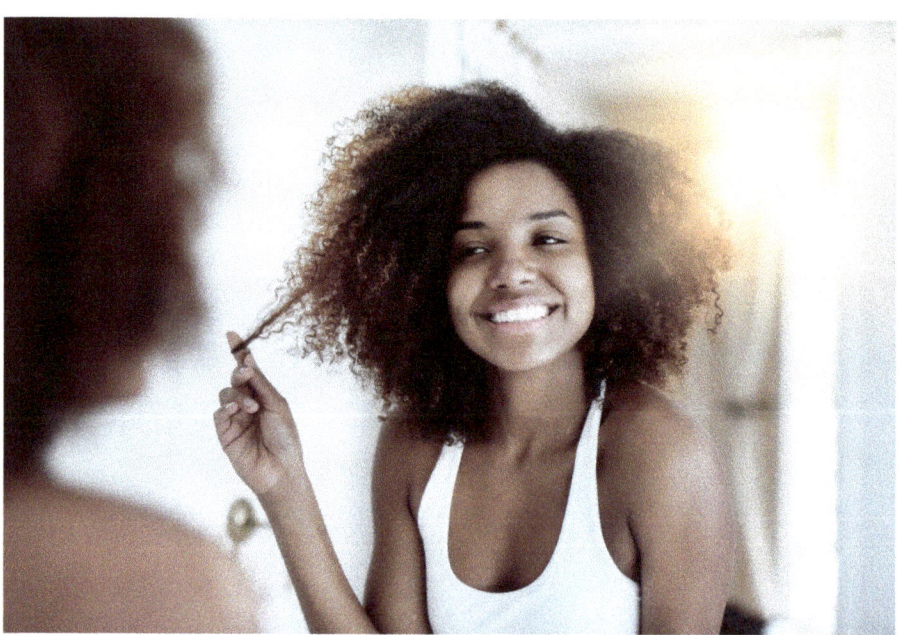

Your Simple 2-Day Hair Care Routine

Day 1: Reset & Protect (Sunday or Your Free Day)

• Deep Condition: Apply a rich conditioning mask (like one with argan or coconut oil). Let it sit for 20-30 minutes, rinse, and follow with a scalp massage to boost growth

• Trim Before Styling: If needed, dust your ends to keep your hair healthy and prevent breakage.

• Protective Style: Opt for twists, braids, or a bun to minimize daily manipulation and protect your hair for the week.

Day 2: Midweek Refresh (Only If Not in a Protective Style)

Co-Wash: Cleanse with a co-wash to hydrate and refresh your hair.
• Moisturize & Seal: Apply a leave-in conditioner, then lock in moisture with a light oil like jojoba or castor oil.

Daily Maintenance
• Spritz dry spots with a water-based moisturizer as needed and always sleep with a satin scarf or on a silk pillowcase.

This routine keeps it quick and easy while ensuring your hair stays healthy, nourished, and ready to thrive!

How Often Should You Wash Your Hair?

Determining the ideal hair-washing frequency can be a bit of a puzzle, but it's all about understanding your hair's unique needs. Factors like hair type, lifestyle, and the products you use play significant roles.

General Guidelines:

- Oily Scalp or Fine Hair: If your scalp tends to get oily or you have fine hair, washing every other day might be beneficial to keep your hair feeling fresh.
- Dry or Coarse Hair: For those with drier hair types, extending the time between washes to once a week or even every two weeks can help maintain natural oils and prevent dryness.
- Active Lifestyle: If you're hitting the gym regularly or engaging in activities that cause sweating, you might find the need to wash your hair more frequently to keep your scalp clean.

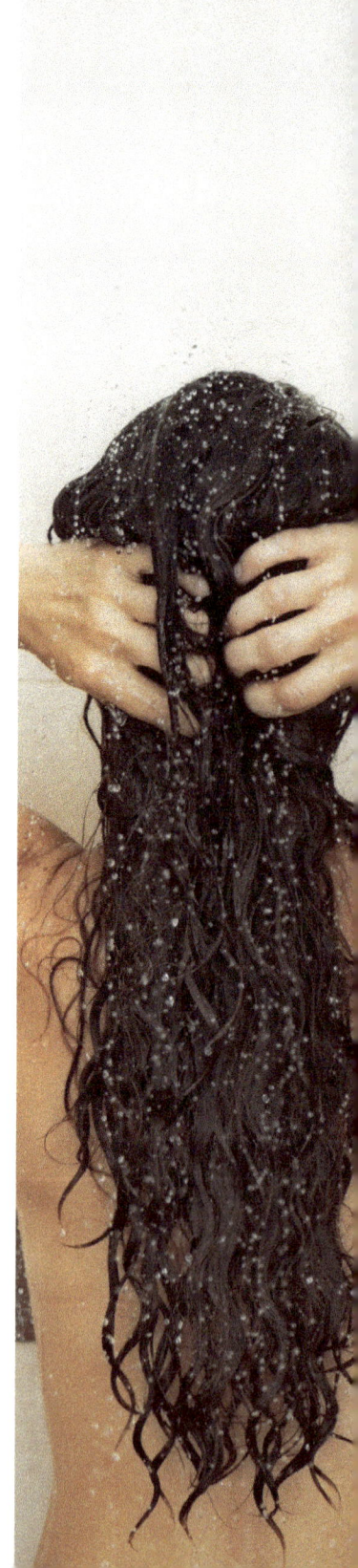

7

Chapter

SCALP TREATMENT

SCALP GOALS

Scalp Check: The Root of It All

Before we get into these DIY scalp treatments, let's talk about the foundation of it all—your scalp. Think of it as the soil in a garden: if it's dry, clogged, or flaky, how do you expect anything to flourish? Whether you're dealing with buildup, itchiness, or just want to give your scalp some extra love, these treatments will help get things back in balance. Because let's be real—healthy hair starts at the root, and your scalp deserves just as much attention as the strands you obsess over. Now, let's get into these easy, effective, and budget-friendly scalp fixes!

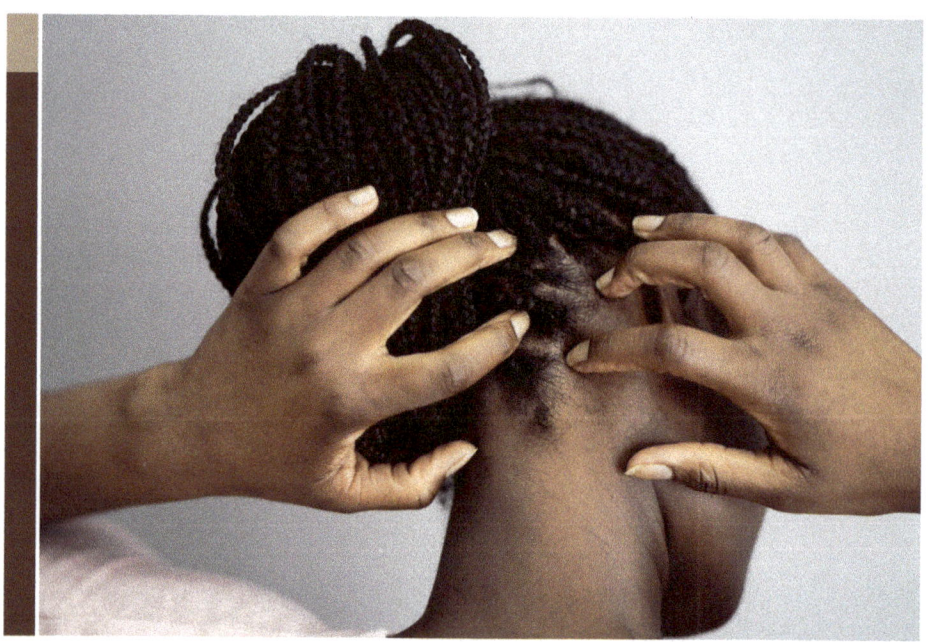

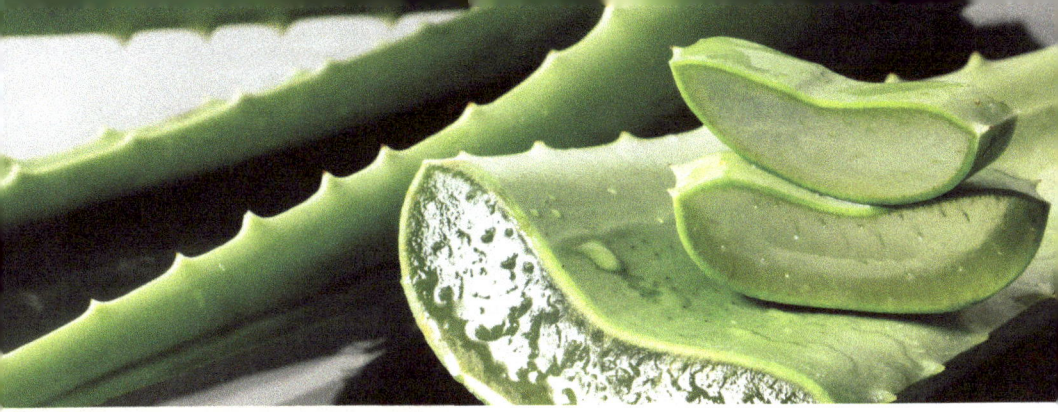

Pre-Treatment: Scalp Detoxifying Mask

Your Best for Texture: All textures (especially beneficial for 3A-4C hair).

Treatment Type: Scalp and hair detox.

INGREDIENTS

1• 2 tbsp bentonite clay

• 1 tbsp apple cider vinegar

• 2 tbsp aloe vera gel

• 1 tbsp jojoba oil

• 1 tsp tea tree essential oil (optional, for dandruff or scalp irritation)

• 2 tbsp water (adjust for consistency)

NOTES

• Shelf Life and Storage: Use immediately. Do not store.
• Benefits: Removes buildup, balances scalp pH, hydrates hair, and strengthens strands for sew-in preparation.

DIRECTIONS

1. In a plastic bowl, mix bentonite clay with water and apple cider vinegar until smooth.

2. Add aloe vera gel, jojoba oil, and tea tree oil. Stir well.

3. Section hair and apply the mask to the scalp and hair (avoid extensions if this is for a re-install).

4. Let sit for 20 minutes. Do not allow it to dry completely.

5. Rinse thoroughly with warm water and follow up with a gentle shampoo.

Scalp Therapy

THE ROOT
OF IT ALL

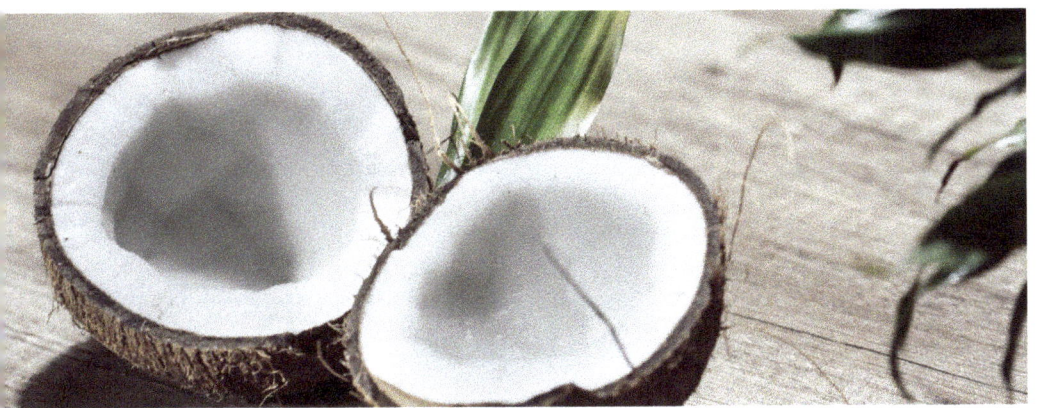

Aloe Glow Up

NOURISHING SCALP SERUM

BEST FOR: ALL HAIR TEXTURES (SOOTHES DRYNESS AND IRRITATION WHILE PROMOTING SCALP HEALTH).

Ingredients

- -2 tablespoons aloe vera gel (pure and unscented)
- - 1 teaspoon coconut oil (liquid form or melted)
- - 3 drops lavender essential oil (optional for soothing)

Directions

1. Mix all ingredients in a small bowl or bottle until well combined.
2. Apply a small amount directly to the scalp using a clean applicator or your fingertips.
3. Massage gently to distribute evenly, focusing on dry areas

This serum can be left in your hair. No rinsing is needed.
Use 2-3 times per week or as needed when your scalp feels dry or irritated.
Shelf Life: 7-10 days in the refrigerator due to aloe vera.

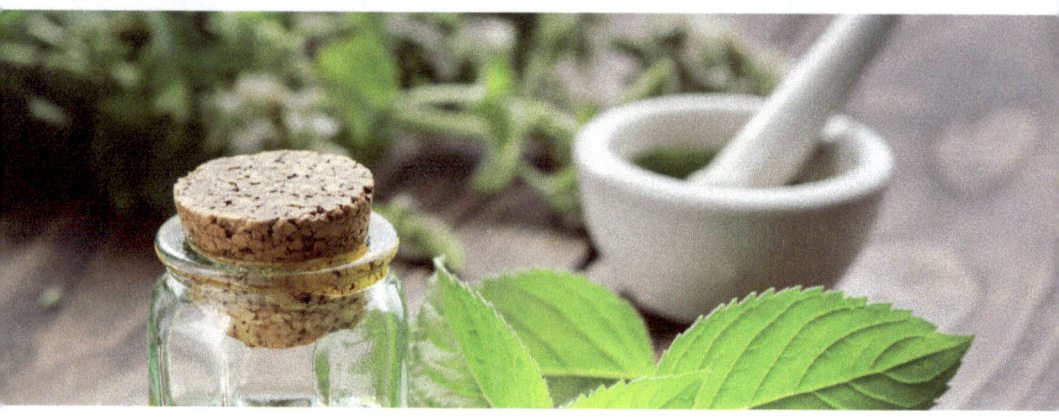

Mint Condition Scalp Mask

BEST FOR: DRY, FLAKY SCALPS (SOOTHES IRRITATION AND PROMOTES CIRCULATION).

Ingredients

- 2 tablespoons plain yogurt
- 1 teaspoon honey
- 3 drops peppermint essential oil

Directions

1. Mix all ingredients into a paste.
2. Apply to your scalp in sections and let sit for 10 minutes.
3. Rinse thoroughly with warm water.

Rinse it out. Use once a week.
Shelf Life: Use immediately, and discard immediately

8

Chapter

GROWTH
RETENTION

GROWTH RETENTION:
KEEPING WHAT YOU GROW

We all love seeing new growth, but the real challenge? Keeping it. What's the point of growing inches if they break off faster than they sprout? Retaining length is all about smart care—hydration, protection, and giving your hair what it needs to thrive. In this chapter, we're focusing on strengthening those strands from root to tip, so all your hard work doesn't go to waste. And of course, I've got a powerhouse DIY recipe to help you lock in that growth. Let's get into it!

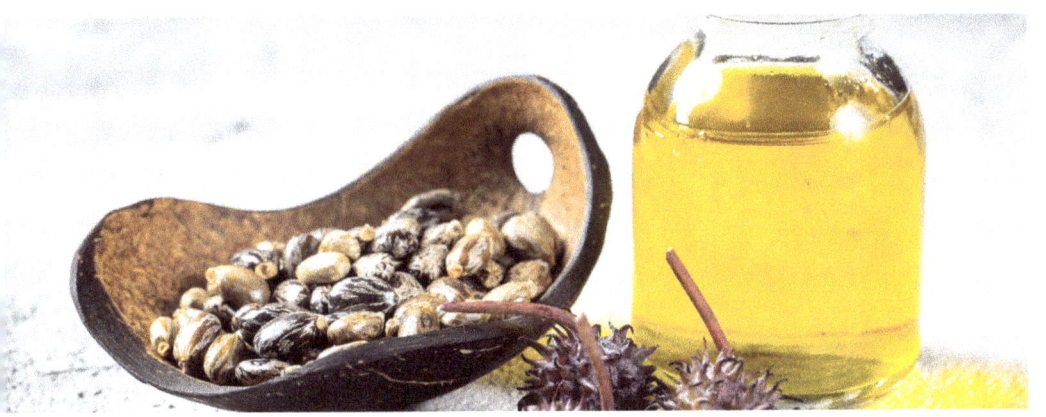

Thick & Thriving

HAIR GROWTH MASK

BEST FOR: STIMULATING OVERALL HAIR GROWTH.

Ingredients

- 2 tablespoons ground flaxseeds (soaked in water for 30 minutes)
- 1 tablespoon coconut oil
- 1 teaspoon castor oil

Directions

1. Blend ingredients into a smooth paste.
2. Apply to the scalp and massage gently.
3. Leave for 30 minutes, then rinse thoroughly.

Use Immediately Do Not Store

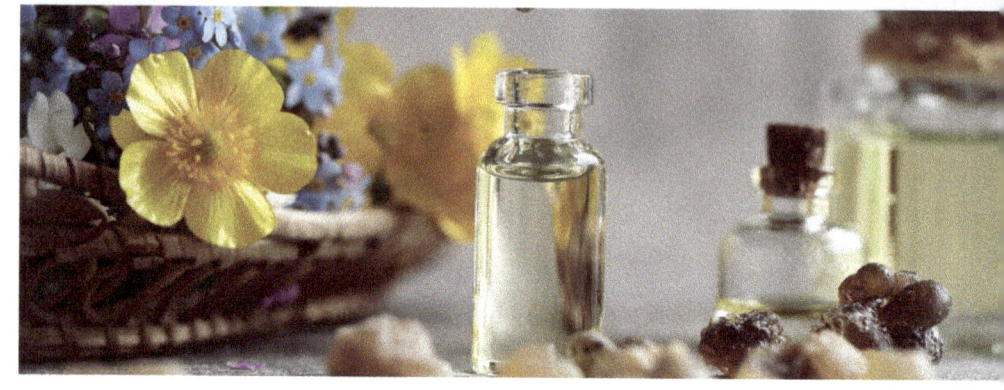

Edge Revival Balm

STRENGTHING BALM FOR THINNING EDGES

BEST FOR: STIMULATING OVERALL HAIR GROWTH.

Ingredients

- 2 tablespoons castor oil
- 1 teaspoon peppermint essential oil
- 1 capsule vitamin E oil (or 1/2 teaspoon liquid vitamin E)

Directions

1. In a small glass bowl, combine castor oil and aloe vera gel.
2. Add peppermint essential oil and vitamin E oil. Mix thoroughly until smooth.
3. Transfer the mixture to a small, airtight container (e.g., a cosmetic jar).
4. Store in a cool, dry place away from sunlight to maintain potency

Recommended Hair Types:
• *Suitable for all hair types, particularly fragile or thinning edges common in Type 3 and 4 hair.*
Frequency of Use:
• *Apply nightly before bed. Use clean hands or a soft applicator brush to gently massage the balm into thinning edges.*

9

Chapter

STYLE CHRONICLES

HAIR HUSTLE HACKS:
QUICK TIPS FOR EVERY STYLE

Sis, we try it all—braids, weaves, blowouts, and color. But let's be real, every style comes with its own set of dos and don'ts. Whether you're protecting your edges, maintaining moisture, or making sure that lace stays flawless, I've got you covered. Here's your go-to cheat sheet for keeping your hair thriving through it all.

▶ Braids & Protective Styles: Keep Your Edges, Sis!

Braids are cute, but traction alopecia? Not so much. Here's how to slay safely:

- Speak Up! If your braids are too tight, say something. A style that lasts four months isn't worth missing your edges for life.
- Moisturize Like You Mean It. Don't just oil your scalp—work that hydration down the braids to keep your strands nourished from root to tip.
- Avoid Heavy Styles. Extra-long or super-thick braids can put too much tension on your scalp.
- Sleep Smart. A satin or silk scarf helps keep your braids looking fresh without unnecessary friction.
- Wash & Refresh. Cleanse your scalp every 2-3 weeks with a diluted shampoo or scalp mist to avoid buildup and itchiness.

> **Pro Tip:** Apply a lightweight leave-in conditioner to your braids to keep them soft and avoid breakage when taking them out.

Underneath it All

RECIPES FOR SEW-IN & WIGS

SEW-IN SECRETS: KEEP IT CUTE, KEEP IT HEALTHY"

We know sew-ins and weaves are the ultimate go-to for slaying any look, but what's really happening underneath? This chapter is packed with fun, easy recipes to keep your scalp fresh and your natural hair moisturized while you rock that protective style. Let's make sure your hair is thriving under there because healthy strands are always in style!

Pro Tips to Keep Your Hair Flourishing:
1. Oil Up, Buttercup: Massage your scalp with a lightweight oil like peppermint or tea tree to keep it fresh and moisturized.

2. Hydrate, Don't Hibernate: A quick spritz of aloe vera and rose water will lock in moisture without messing up your style.

3. Wrap It Right, Keep It Tight: Satin scarves and pillowcases are lifesavers for avoiding friction and keeping your sew-in looking flawless.

4. Keep It Fresh, Babe: Banish buildup with a gentle apple cider vinegar rinse to keep your scalp clean and happy.

With these tips and recipes, your hair will be living its best life, even in a sew-in!
on and take that weave down with hair that's stronger than ever!

Pro Tip:

After removing your quick weave, do a deep conditioning treatment to restore moisture and elasticity.

LACE FRONT WIGS: SLAY SMART, NOT HARD

Lace fronts are life, but sis, they're temporary, not a lifestyle. If you're wearing lace back-to-back, it's time for a break.

- Give Your Hair a Breather. Take breaks between installs to prevent thinning edges and allow your scalp to breathe.
- Scalp Check-Ups. Do regular scalp analyses to monitor for irritation, buildup, or thinning.
- Avoid Excessive Glue. Too much adhesive can cause breakage and bald spots–opt for glueless methods when possible.
- Secure Properly. If you're using glue, ensure it's applied and removed correctly to avoid pulling out your natural hair.
- Edge Protection 101. Use an edge protector underneath your wig to safeguard your hairline.

"

Pro Tip: If you're reapplying your wig often, make sure to cleanse your scalp thoroughly to avoid product buildup and clogged follicles.

"

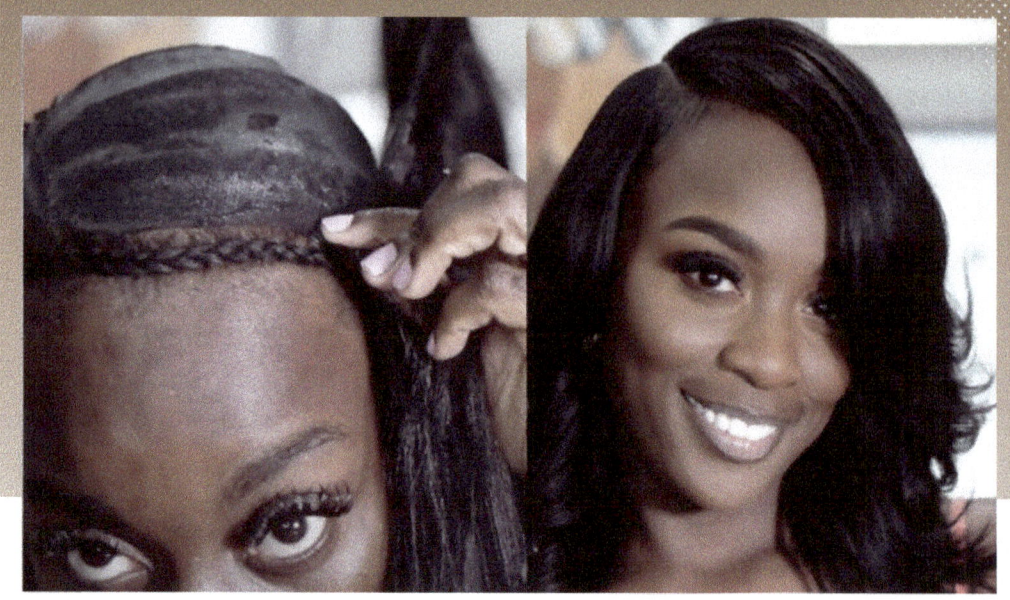

QUICK WEAVES:
FROM GLUE TO GLAM WITHOUT THE DAMAGE

Quick weaves are making a comeback, and thankfully, they're not as risky as they once were—if you do them right.

- Ask Your Stylist About Protection. Before booking, make sure your stylist uses a protective barrier (like liquid caps) to safeguard your natural hair.
- Use a Stocking Cap. This adds an extra layer of protection to prevent glue from getting directly on your hair.
- Proper Removal is Everything. Never rip off a quick weave! Use an oil-based remover or wash with a moisturizing shampoo to break down the glue safely.
- Limit the Heat. Excessive flat ironing on glued-in hair can lead to tangling and damage.
- Hydration Matters. Even under a weave, your hair still needs moisture—don't neglect it.

Refresh & Flex

Scalp Refreshing Cooling Mist

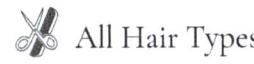 All Hair Types

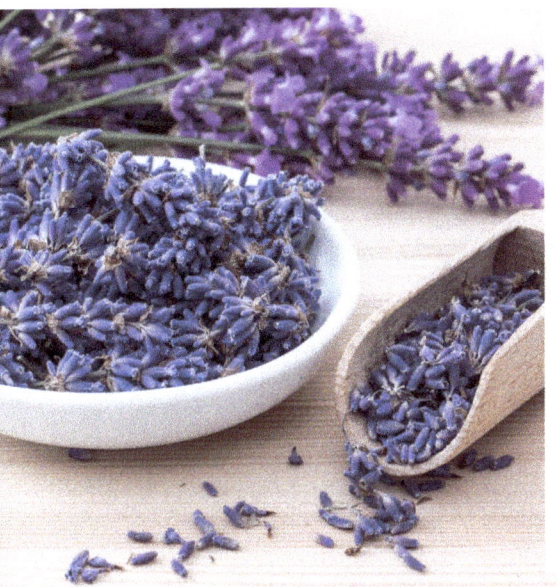

INGREDIENTS

- 1 cup distilled water
- 1 tablespoon aloe vera gel
- 5 drops tea tree essential oil (optional for anti-itch)
- 5 drops lavender essential oil (optional for soothing)

DIRECTIONS

1. Mix all ingredients in a spray bottle and shake well.
2. Section your weave or wig to expose the scalp, and spritz lightly.
3. Massage gently to distribute.

Shelf Life: 7-10 days in the refrigerator (due to aloe vera).

NOTES

Leave it in—no rinsing needed. Use daily or whenever your scalp feels itchy or dry.

Shelf Life: 7-10 days in the refrigerator (due to aloe vera).

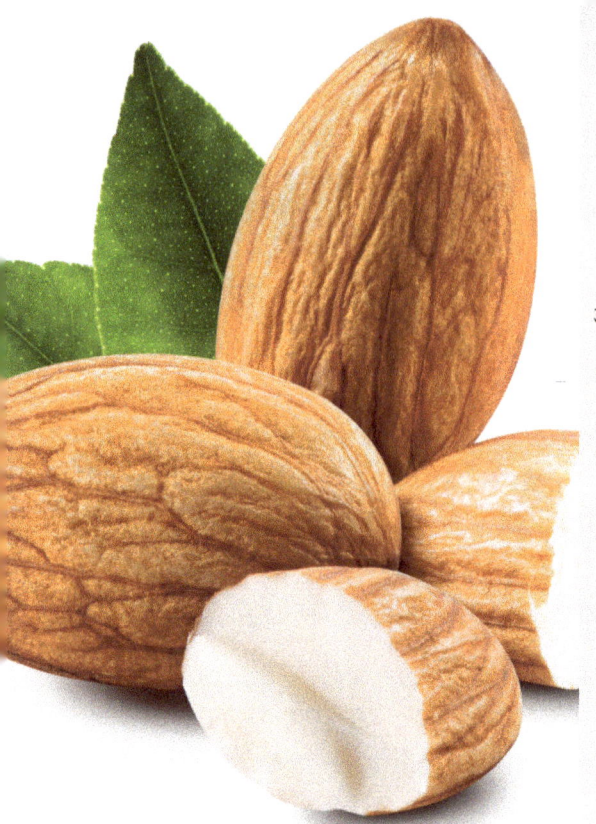

Leave-Out Treatment: Moisturizing and Sealing Cre

3A-4C hair (works well for high-heat protection).

INGREDIENTS

2 tbsp shea butter (melted)
• 1 tbsp sweet almond oil
• 1 tbsp aloe vera gel
• 1 tsp argan oil
• 1 tsp glycerin
• 5 drops rosemary essential oil (optional, for growth)

DIRECTIONS

1. In a bowl, mix melted shea butter with sweet almond oil, argan oil, and aloe vera gel.
 2. Add glycerin and rosemary oil (if using). Stir until creamy.
3. Apply a small amount to leave-out hair after styling or when dry.
4. Use sparingly to avoid weighing down the hair.

NOTES
• Shelf Life and Storage: Store in a cool, dry place for up to 3 months.
• Benefits: Hydrates dry hair, adds shine, protects from heat, and strengthens strands to prevent breakage.

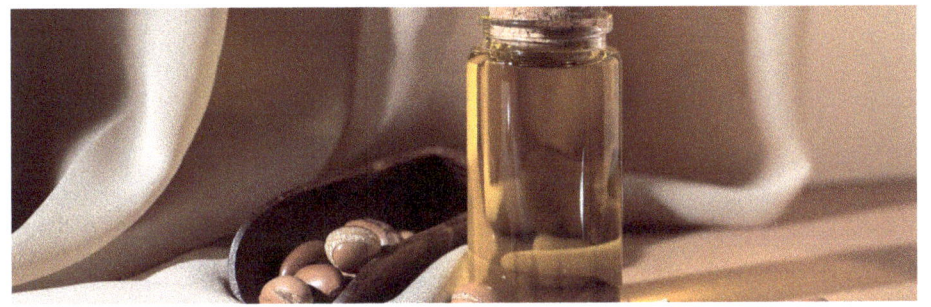

Milky Way Mist

LEAVE OUT HYDRATION MOISTURE SPRAY
BEST FOR: STRAIGHT, WAVY, AND CURLY TEXTURES (PROVIDES HYDRATION
AND SHINE FOR LEAVE-OUT SECTIONS).

Ingredients

- 1/2 cup distilled water
• 1/4 cup coconut milk (available in cans at grocery stores)
• 1 teaspoon argan oil (or olive oil)

Directions

1. Mix all ingredients in a small bowl or bottle until well combined.
2. Apply a small amount directly to the scalp using a clean applicator or your fingertips.
3. Massage gently to distribute evenly, focusing on dry areas.

This spray is a leave-in. No rinsing required.
Use daily or every other day for soft, hydrated, and frizz-free leave-out.
Shelf Life: 5-7 days in the refrigerator (shake before each use).

Wig Whisper

Under-Wig Scalp Spray

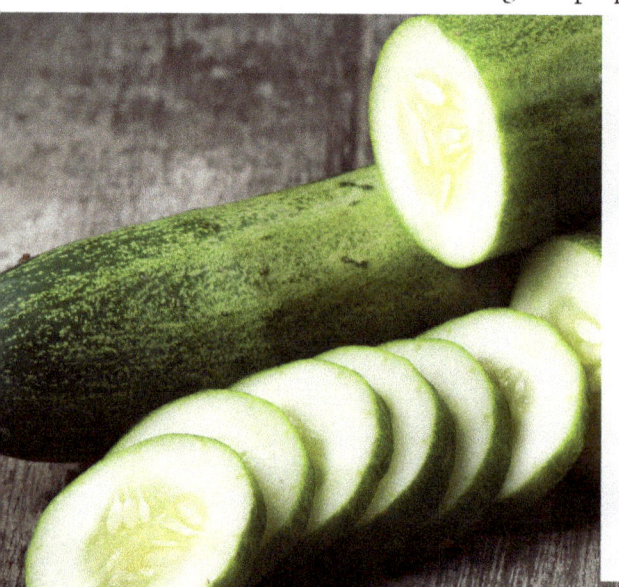

 Wigs or Weaves

INGREDIENTS

1/2 cup distilled water
• 1 teaspoon tea tree oil
• 1 teaspoon Aloe Vera Gel or Cucumber Gel

DIRECTIONS

1. Mix all ingredients in a spray bottle and shake well.
2. Section your weave or wig to expose the scalp, and spritz lightly.
3. Massage gently to distribute.

NOTES

Best For: Reducing dryness and itchiness under wigs. Shelf Life: store in the refrigerator due to aloe vera Up to 1 month in a cool, dry place.

Slay it Straight

THE SILK PRESS SURVIVAL GUIDE

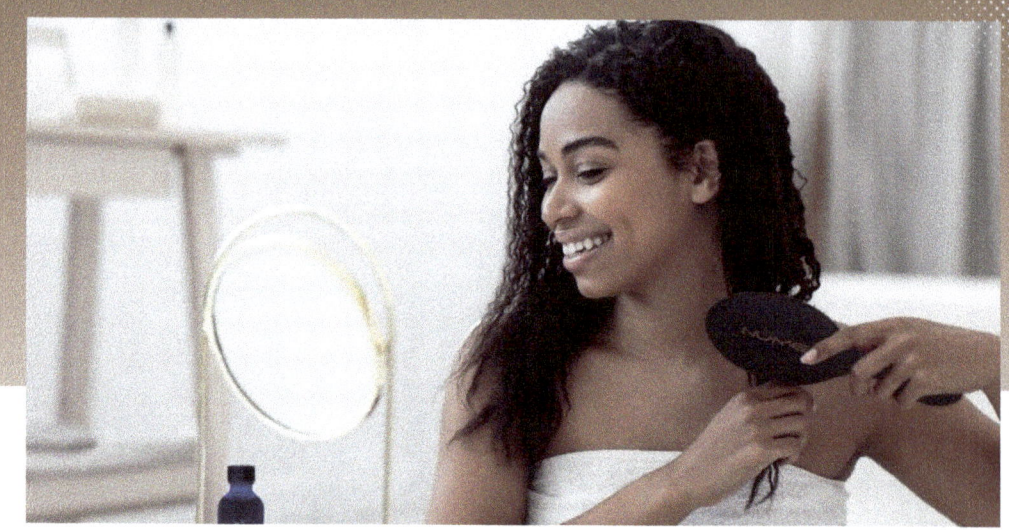

SILK PRESSES & BLOWOUTS:
KEEP THE HEAT IN CHECK

A sleek silk press is everything, but too much heat? That's a curl killer. Here's how to keep your bounce:

- Hydration is Key. In between presses, treat your hair to deep hydration masks to keep it healthy and bouncy.
- Protect Your Curl Pattern. Limit heat usage to every 2-3 weeks max to prevent heat damage.
- Use a Heat Protectant. Always apply a thermal protectant before styling–no excuses.
- Avoid Excessive Straightening. If your hair starts to feel stiff and brittle, it's time to back off the heat.
- Wrap it Right. Use silk or satin wraps to keep your press looking fresh without needing touch-ups.

> **Pro Tip:** If you notice your curls aren't bouncing back, it might be time to give heat a break and focus on restoring elasticity.

Silky Smooth Spray

Moisturizer

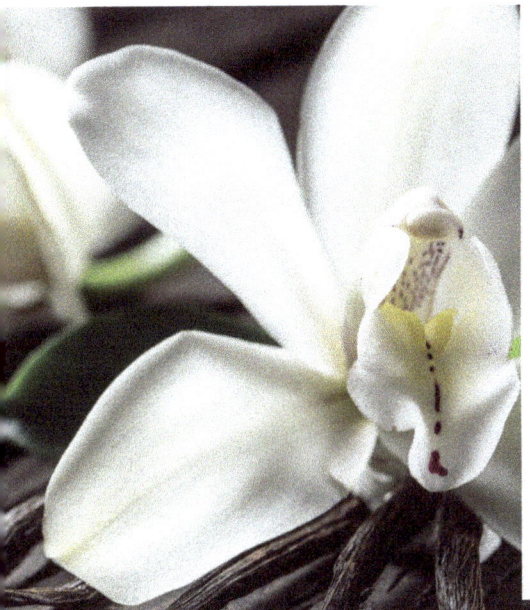

INGREDIENTS

 All Hair Types

• 1/4 cup aloe vera juice
• 1/4 cup distilled water
• 1 tablespoon argan oil
• 2 drops vanilla essential oil (optional for a sweet scent)

DIRECTIONS

1. Combine all ingredients in a spray bottle and shake well.
2. Lightly mist your hair before or after styling to lock in moisture and add shine.

Best For: Straight and wavy textures (protects hair while adding hydration). Leave it in. Use daily or as needed for hydration.

NOTES

Shelf Life: 5-7 days in the refrigerator.

Press & Protect Potion

Silk Press Heat Protection Spray

INGREDIENTS

- 1/2 cup distilled water
- 1 tablespoon argan oil
- 1 teaspoon aloe vera gel
- 5 drops grapeseed oil

DIRECTIONS

Mix all ingredients in a spray bottle. Lightly mist onto damp hair before blow-drying or flat ironing.

NOTES

Protecting natural hair from heat damage during silk presses.

- Leave-in or rinse? Leave it in. Shelf Life: Up to 1 month.

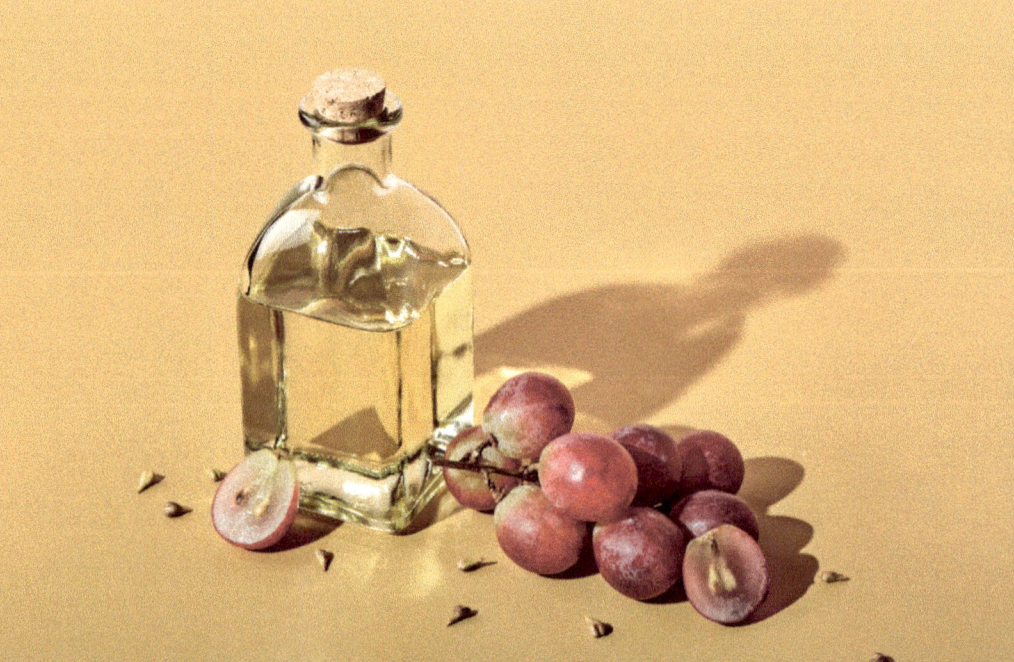

Sleek Chic Serum

Post-Silk Press Maintenance

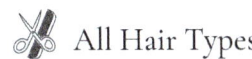 All Hair Types

INGREDIENTS

1 tablespoon jojoba oil
- 1 teaspoon vitamin E oil
- 3 drops lavender essential oil

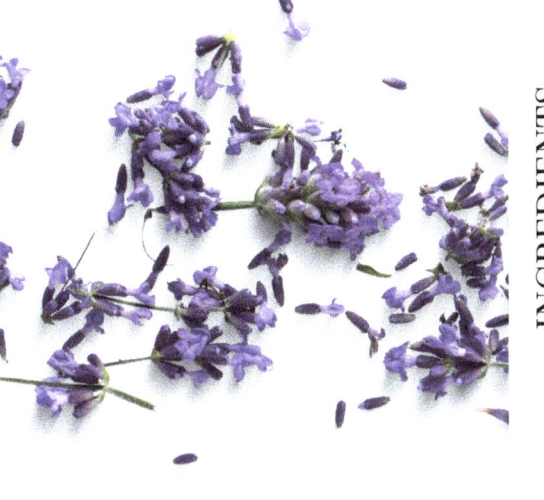

DIRECTIONS

Apply a small amount to hands and smooth over hair, focusing on ends.

Maintaining shine and reducing frizz after heat styling.

NOTES

Leave it in—no rinsing needed. Use daily or whenever needed

Shelf Life: 6 months

CURL CHRONICLES

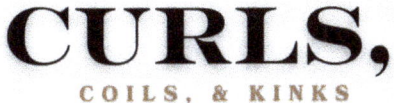

CURLS,
COILS, & KINKS

Moisture is the secret sauce to juicy, defined curls –because the drier the hair, the duller the vibe. The key? Hydration + protection = length retention. If your curls are feeling like tumbleweed instead of springy spirals, it's time to turn up the moisture!

DO:

✓ Warm up your moisturizer or oil–because hair loves a little heat (the good kind).

✓ Seal it in with a butter or oil so your hair stays quenched, not thirsty.

✓ Detangle like you love your hair, not like you're mad at it.

DON'T:

✗ Skip deep conditioning unless you like crunchy curls.

✗ Overdo it with heavy products–build-up is not a look.

✗ Ignore your ends! Retention is about keeping what you grow, not watching it snap off.

Now, let's get into this recipe–because your curls deserve to be soft, bouncy, and living their best life!

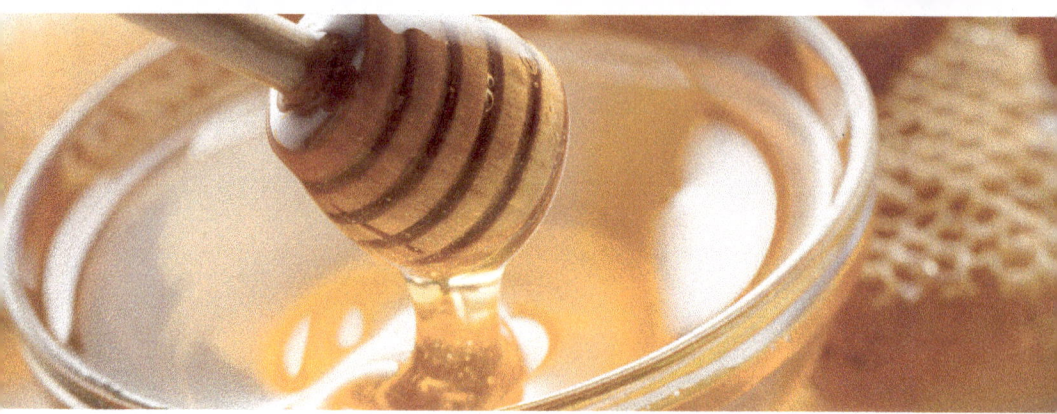

Curl Power

DEFINING CURLY GEL

BEST FOR: 3A TO 4C CURLS (FOR DEFINITION AND FRIZZ CONTROL).

Ingredients

- 2 tablespoons flaxseeds
- 1 cup distilled water
- 1 teaspoon honey
- 3 drops lavender
essential oil

Directions

1. Boil flaxseeds in water for 5 minutes. Strain the gel-like liquid into a bowl.
2. Stir in honey and essential oil.
3. Let cool, then store in a jar.

Leave it in for defined, bouncy curls. Use after every wash or whenever styling.
Shelf Life: 7-10 days in the refrigerator.

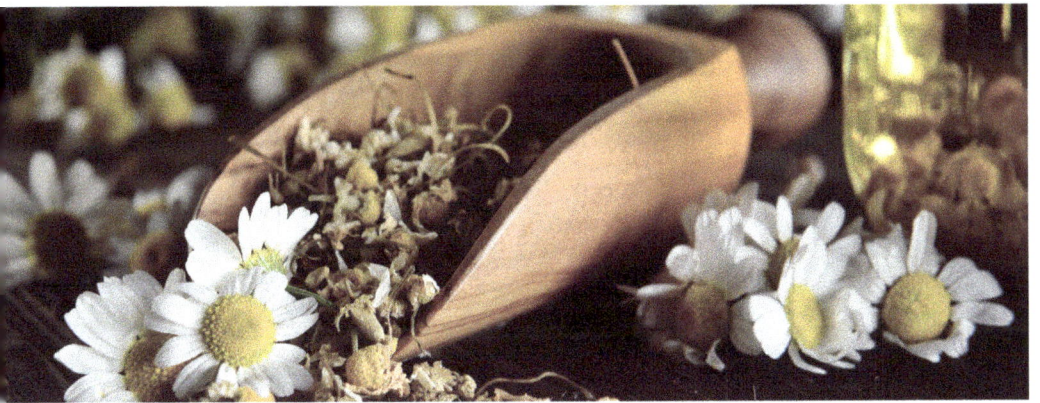

Knot Today Spray

DETANGLING SPRAY

✔ CURLY (3A–3C) & COILY (4A–4C) HAIR:

• HELPS SOFTEN CURLS AND COILS, MAKING DETANGLING EASIER WITH LESS BREAKAGE.

• ADDS MOISTURE AND SLIP, REDUCING KNOTS AND SINGLE-STRAND TANGLES.

Ingredients

- 1 cup distilled water
- 2 tablespoons aloe vera juice
- 1 teaspoon glycerin
- 1 teaspoon jojoba oil
- 5 drops chamomile essential oil
- (gentle & soothing for the scalp)

Directions

1. Mix all ingredients in a spray bottle and shake well.
2. Lightly mist onto damp or dry hair before detangling.
3. Use fingers and or a wide-tooth comb to gently remove knots.

Notes:

Great for refreshing curls between wash days.

• Aloe vera hydrates while glycerin helps attract moisture.

Chamomile soothes the scalp and keeps hair soft.

• Shelf Life: 2 weeks when stored in the fridge.

Tressed to Impress:
THE BRAID EDITION"

PROTECTIVE STYLES:

KEEP IT CUTE, KEEP IT HEALTHY

From Boho Knotless and faux locs to classic cornrows, protective styles are the plug for low-maintenance slayage. But listen—protective doesn't mean neglective. If your scalp is screaming and your braids look like they've seen some things... we've got work to do. This section is all about keeping your styles fresh, your scalp happy, and your hair thriving underneath. No flakes, no itch—just vibes.

DO:
Oil your scalp lightly—greasy braids are not the move.
Wrap it up at night. A bonnet or scarf isn't a suggestion, it's a necessity.
Refresh your roots with a little mist and scalp care to keep the itchies away.

DON'T:
Keep a style in past its expiration date. If it's hanging on for dear life, let it go.
Tug or retighten your edges. Snatched edges today, missing edges tomorrow.
Forget to wash your hair. Sweat, dirt, and buildup don't magically disappear.

Now, let's get into the recipes that'll keep your protective styles looking flawless and your scalp feeling brand new!

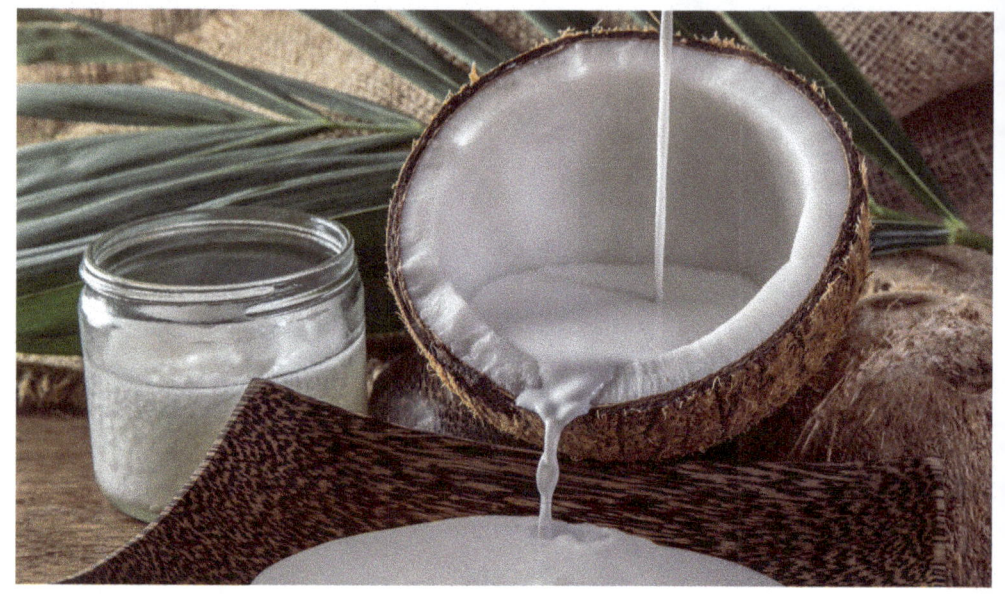

Braid Babe Prep

SCALP HYDRATION OIL

Ingredients

2 tablespoons castor oil

1 tablespoon peppermint oil

1 teaspoon tea tree oil

Directions

Massage into scalp 15 minutes before braiding.

BEST FOR: MOISTURIZING AND PROTECTING THE SCALP BEFORE BRAIDING.

Leave it in. Use after every wash or as needed.
Shelf Life: 3 months in a cool, dry place.

Did you know?

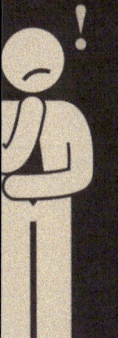

Protective styles like braids and twists can help retain length, but they must be properly maintained to prevent tension damage and breakage.

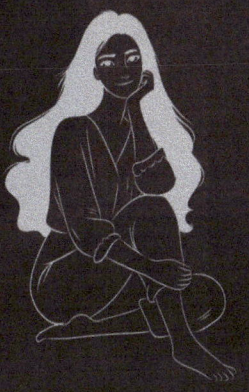

Braid Bomb Refresh Spray

Itch relief & Moisturizing Spray

INGREDIENTS

- 1/2 cup rose water
- 1 tablespoon aloe vera gel
- 5 drops tea tree oil

DIRECTIONS

1. Combine all ingredients in a spray bottle and shake.
2. Spritz onto your scalp and braids for a refreshing boost.

NOTES

Best For: All protective styles (scalp hydration and itch relief).

Leave it in.Use daily to keep your scalp itch-free.

Shelf Life: 7 days in the refrigerator.

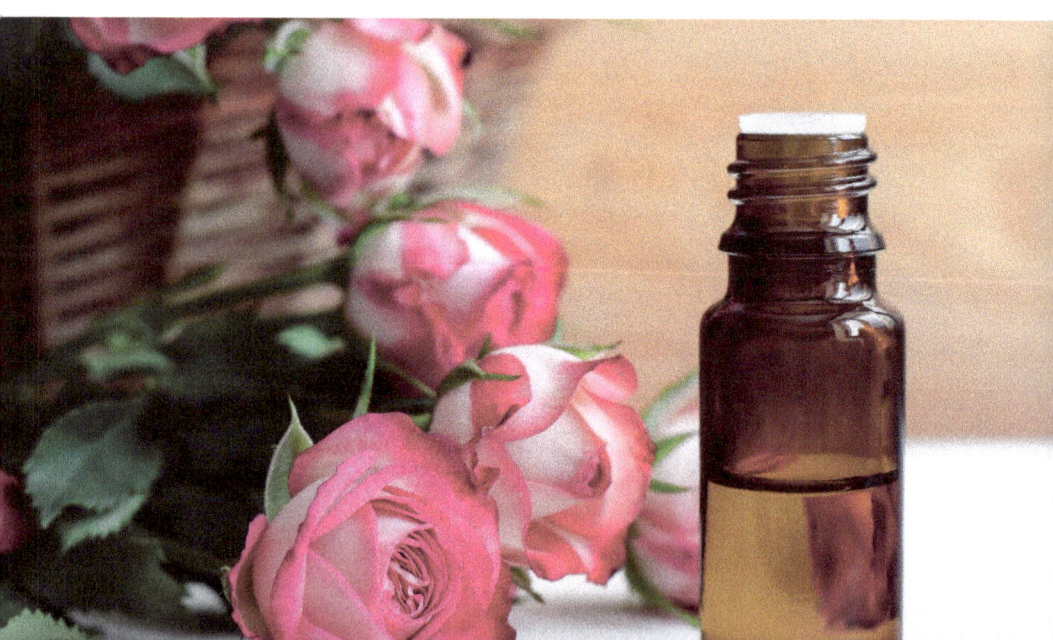

Unravel Me

Post-Braid Detangling Serum

INGREDIENTS

1/4 cup apple cider vinegar
- 1/4 cup water
- 1 teaspoon olive oil

DIRECTIONS

Apply generously to hair before washing to prevent matting and tangles.

NOTES

Best For: Easing detangling after braid removal.

Use immediately; do not store.

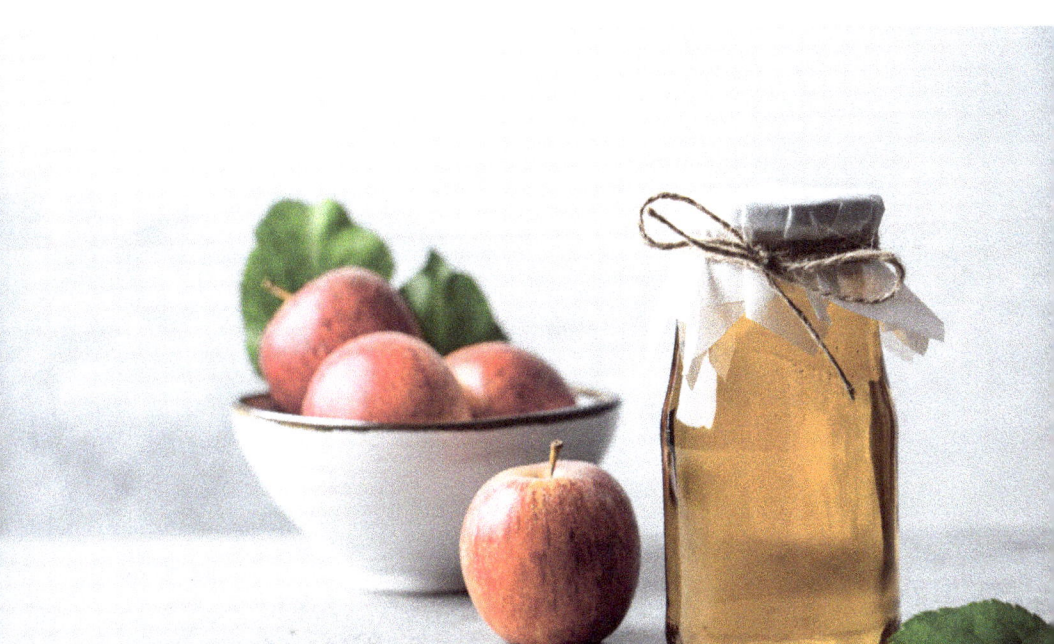

Locked In:

THE ULTIMATE GUIDE TO LOCS & SISTERLOCKS

LOC QUEENS:

Whether you're in the baby loc stage or your locs have seen more birthdays than your little cousin, one thing's for sure–hydration and maintenance are mandatory! Because let's be real, nobody wants crunchy, lint-filled, buildup-packed locs. This section is all about keeping them fresh, flourishing, and free from drama.

DO:
✔ Keep your scalp moisturized–ashy roots are not a personality trait.
✔ Rinse your locs–water won't undo your journey, but product buildup might!
✔ Use lightweight oils and mists–because nobody wants stiff, greasy locs.

DON'T:
✖ Cake on heavy products–your locs aren't a pantry, no need for extra "storage."
✖ Let lint move in rent-free–wrap it up at night like you love your hair.
✖ Retwist every five minutes–edges and scalp need a break too!

Now, let's get into these recipes–because hydrated, healthy locs hit different!

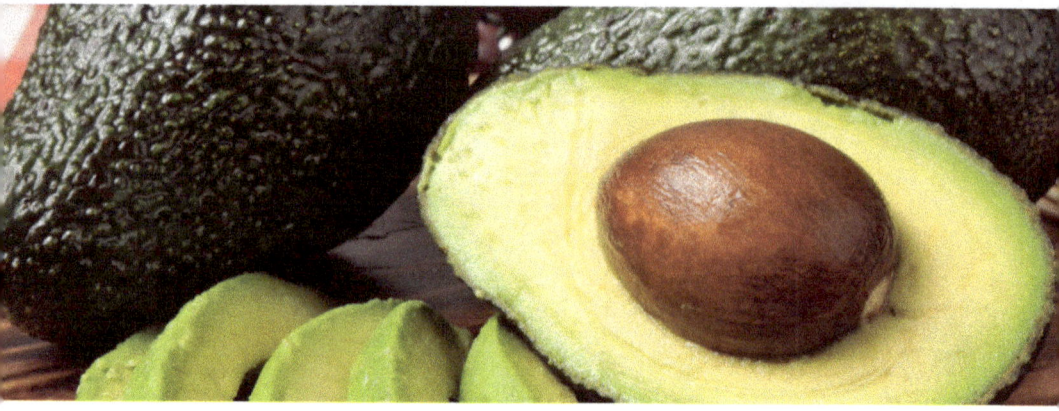

Loc Love Oil

MOISTURIZING OIL

BEST FOR: LOCS AND SISTERLOCKS (ADDS SHINE AND
PREVENTS DRYNESS).

Ingredients

- 2 tablespoons jojoba oil
- 1 tablespoon avocado oil
- 5 drops rosemary
essential oil

Directions

1. Mix in a small bottle.
2. Apply directly to your scalp and the length of your locs.
3. Massage gently to distribute.

Leave it in. Use 1-2 times weekly or as needed.
Shelf Life: 6 months in a cool, dark place.

Other Styles We Love (and Need to Maintain Right!)

Clip-Ins & Tape-Ins:

- Always remove gently to avoid snags and breakage.
- Blend with your natural hair using minimal heat.
- Clean and condition extensions regularly for longevity.

Locs & Sisterlocks:

- Moisturize regularly to prevent brittleness.
- Avoid product buildup with lightweight oils and clarifying washes.
- Retwist on schedule to keep them looking fresh without too much tension.

Bantu Knots & Twist Outs:

- Prep with a moisturizing leave-in for defined, hydrated curls.
- Use satin bonnets overnight to preserve the style.
- Fluff gently with your fingers to avoid frizz.

Final Thoughts: It's All About Balance

No matter your style of choice, the key to thriving hair is balance. Listen to your hair, treat it with love, and make sure you're giving it what it needs—whether that's moisture, protection, or just a break from all the styling. Because let's be real, the best style is healthy hair!

YOUR HAIR
VS
The weather

SEASONAL

YEAR-ROUND HAIRCARE: BECAUSE THE WEATHER STAYS PLAYING GAMES

From winter's ashy, moisture-snatching cold to summer's frizz-inducing humidity, your hair goes through a lot. One season it's begging for hydration, the next it's screaming for protection. But no worries—this section has the recipes to keep your strands thriving no matter what Mother Nature throws your way. Because healthy hair isn't seasonal, it's a lifestyle!

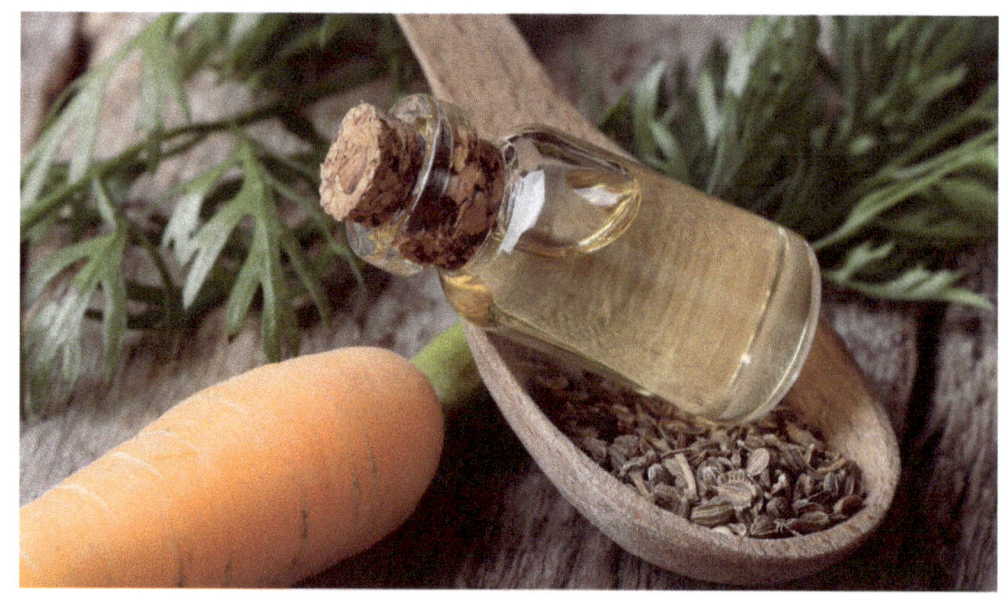

Sunshine Shield Spray

BEST FOR: DRY, FLAKY SCALPS (SOOTHES IRRITATION AND PROMOTES CIRCULATION).

Ingredients

- 1/2 cup green tea (cooled)
- 1 tablespoon aloe vera juice
- 3 drops carrot seed oil

Directions

1. Combine ingredients in a spray bottle and shake.
2. Spritz onto your hair before heading out.

Notes

Leave it in. Use daily in sunny weather.
Shelf Life: 5 days in the refrigerator.

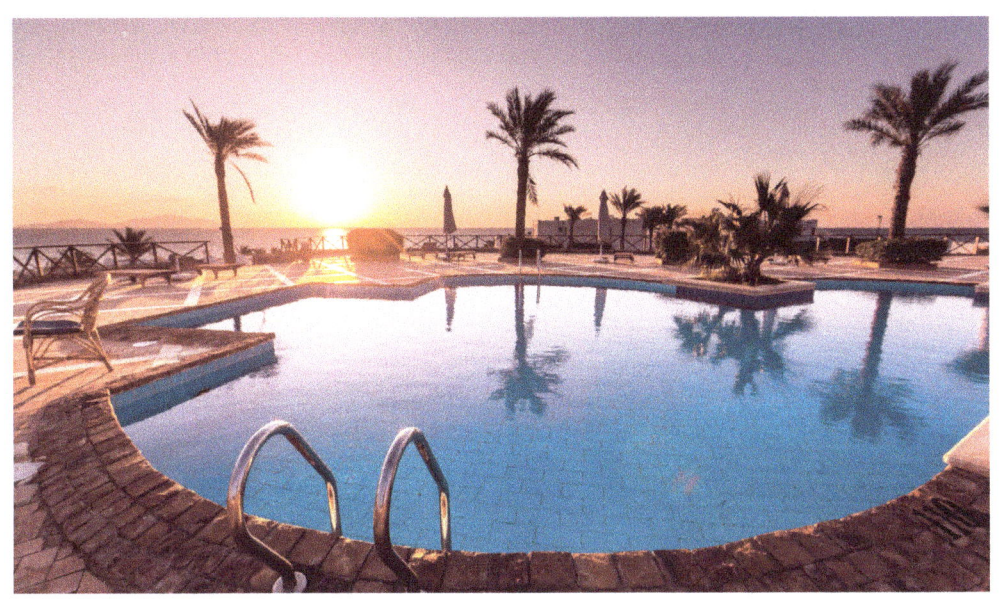

Summer Swimmers' Hair Shield

PROTECTS AGAINST CHLORINE & SUN DAMAGE (BEST FOR SWIMMERS & BEACHGOERS OF ALL HAIR TYPES)

Ingredients

- 2 tablespoons coconut oil
- 1 tablespoon aloe vera gel
- 1 teaspoon jojoba oil
- 1 teaspoon apple cider vinegar
- 5 drops tea tree essential oil

Directions

- Coconut oil helps prevent chlorine absorption.
- Aloe vera soothes sun-exposed hair and scalp.
- Apple cider vinegar helps remove chlorine buildup post-swim.

Notes

Shelf Life: 1 month, store in a cool place.

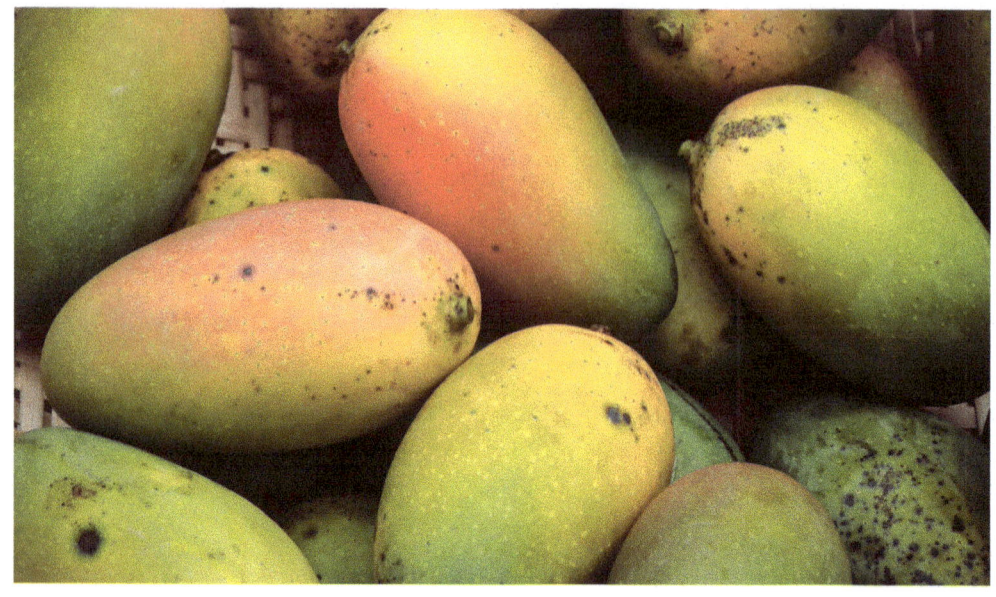

Cold Weather Hydration Butter

FOR DRY, BRITTLE HAIR IN WINTER (BEST FOR ALL HAIR TYPES, ESPECIALLY 3A TO 4C CURLS)

Ingredients

- 2 tablespoons mango butter
- 1 tablespoon avocado oil
- 1 teaspoon castor oil
- 1 teaspoon honey
- 5 drops peppermint essential oil

Directions

1. Melt the mango butter and avocado oil together using a double boiler or microwave in short bursts.
2. Stir in castor oil, honey, and peppermint essential oil.
3. Whip or stir until creamy and smooth.
4. Store in a jar and use as a daily sealant to lock in moisture.

Best used on damp hair after applying a leave-in conditioner.
Helps combat dryness,
breakage, and static caused by cold weather.
• Shelf Life: 2 months in a cool,

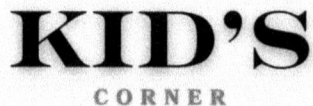

KID'S
CORNER

LITTLE CURLS, BIG CARE: BECAUSE TANGLES AND TEARS ARE NOT ON THE AGENDA

Tiny curls, coils, and kinks deserve big love! Whether your little one's hair is always in motion (just like them) or they're rocking cute protective styles, gentle care is key. No more yanking, no more tears—just soft, hydrated, and tangle-free hair that stays adorable and manageable. These recipes are made to keep their strands thriving without the drama, because wash day should be fun (or at least less stressful).

Now, let's get into these kid-friendly, fuss-free formulas!

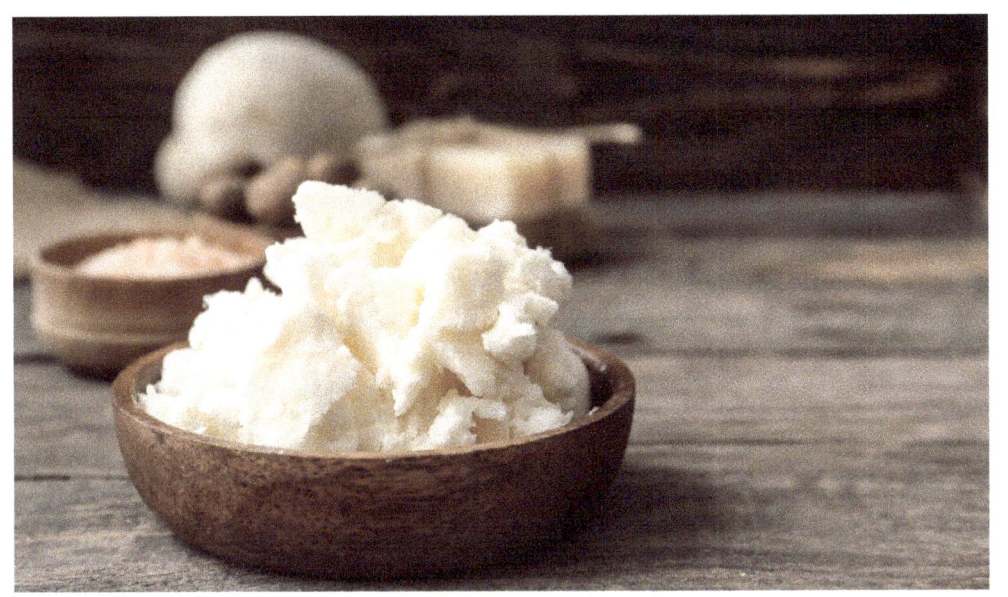

DewYou Boo

FOR HYDRATED, DEFINED CURLS (BEST FOR 3A TO 4C HAIR)

Ingredients

- 1/4 cup shea butter
- 1 teaspoon olive oil
- 1 teaspoon coconut oil

Directions

1. Melt shea butter and mix with oils.
2. Let cool and whip into a creamy texture.
3. Apply a small amount to damp hair and style as desired.

Apply to damp curls after washing for hydration and definition.• Works great as a leave-in or twist-out cream. • Shelf Life: 2-3 weeks when stored in a cool, dry place.

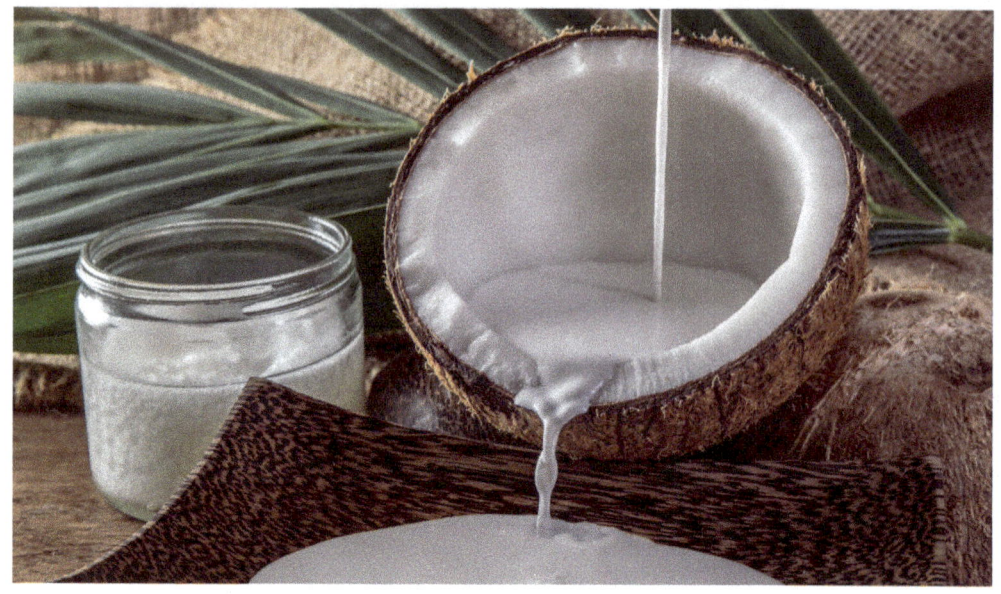

Kiddie Curl Cream

BEST FOR: SOFT CURLS AND COILS (DETANGLES AND DEFINES).

Ingredients

- 2 tablespoons shea butter
- 1 tablespoon coconut oil
- 1 tablespoon aloe vera gel
- 1 teaspoon honey
- 5 drops rosemary essential oil

Directions

1. Melt the shea butter and coconut oil together using a double boiler or microwave (short intervals).2. Let it cool slightly, then mix in aloe vera gel, honey, and rosemary essential oil.3. Whip or stir until creamy.4. Store in a jar and use as a curl-defining cream on damp hair.

Leave it in. Use after every wash or as needed.
Shelf Life: 6 months in a cool, dry place.

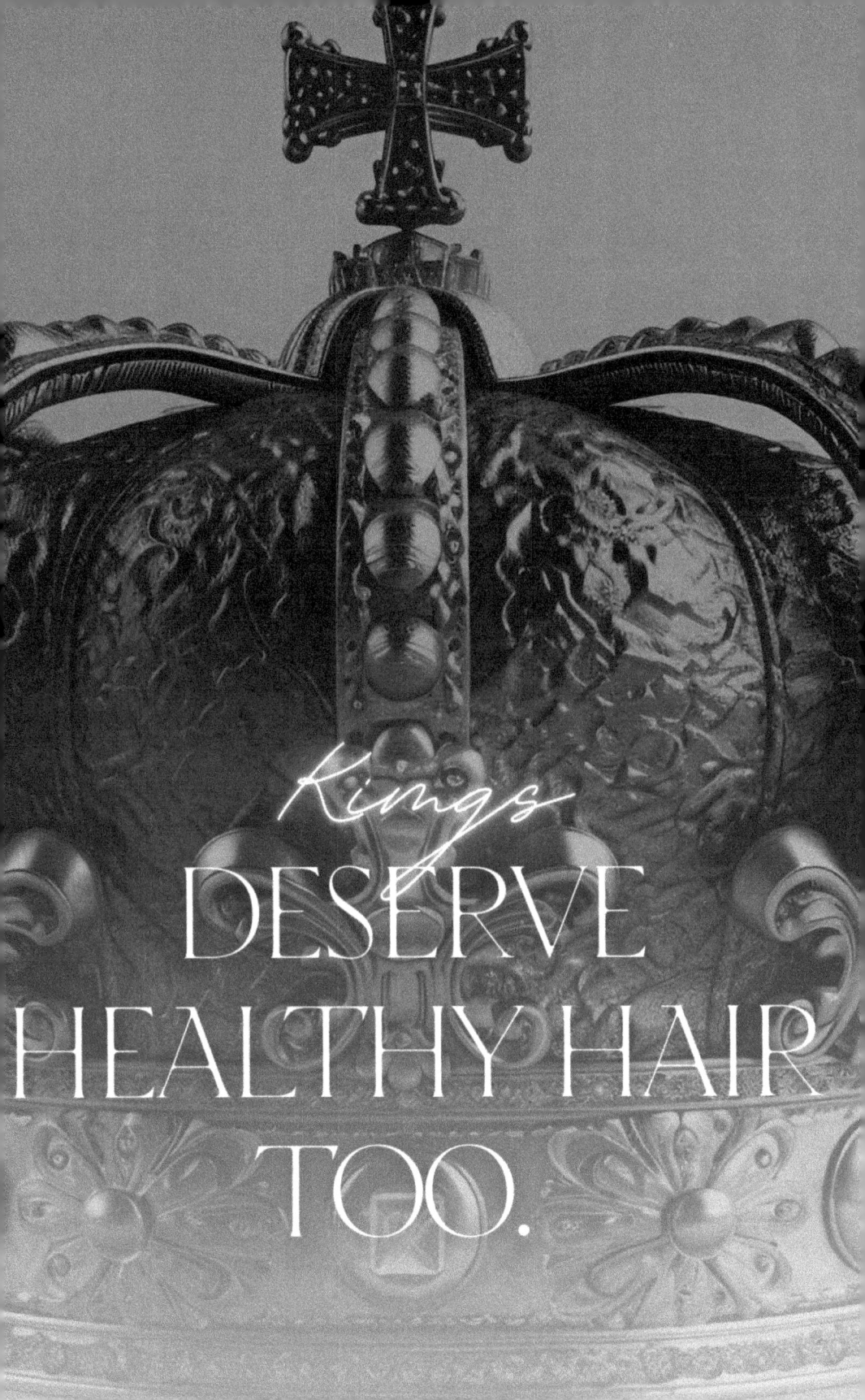

KINGS

DESERVES HEALTHY HAIR TOO

Fellas, hair care isn't just for the ladies—your crown deserves attention too! Whether you're dealing with thinning, dryness, or just want your waves, curls, or locs to stay fresh, these recipes are here to level up your routine. No fluff, no complicated steps—just effective, easy-to-use treatments to keep your hair and scalp thriving. Because real kings take care of their crowns!

Crown King

Men's Oil for Thinning Hair

INGREDIENTS

- 2 tablespoons castor oil
- 1 teaspoon black seed oil
- 1 teaspoon peppermint oil

DIRECTIONS

Massage into scalp for 5 minutes nightly. Leave overnight and rinse in the morning.

NOTES

Best For: Stimulating hair growth in men..

Shelf Life: Up to 6 months. use daily.

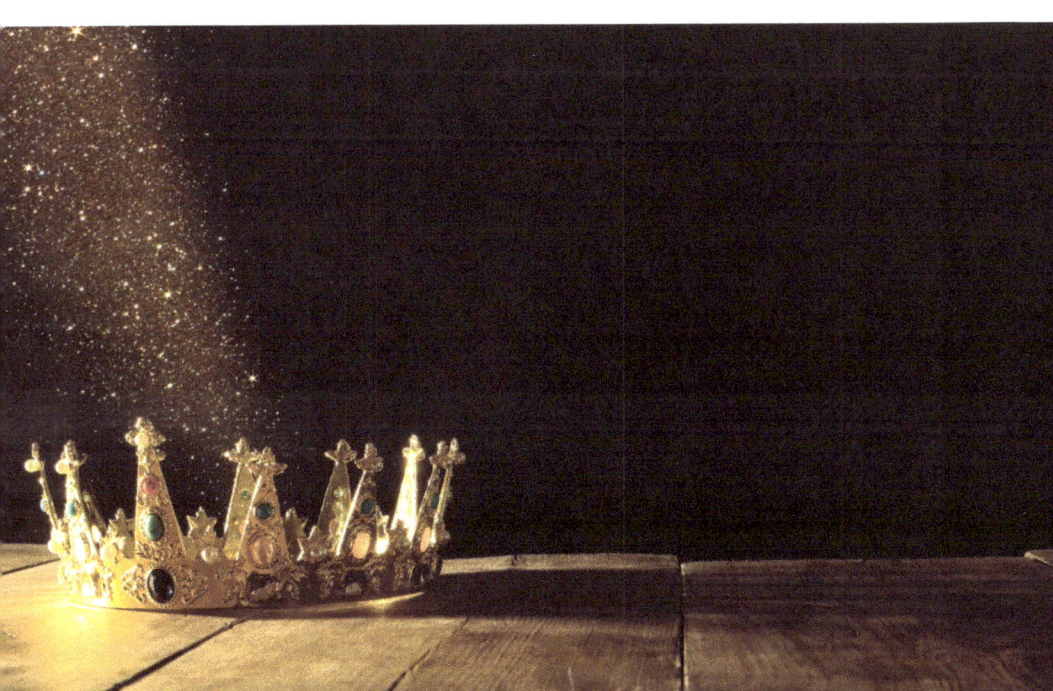

Mommy Mant

POSTPARTUM HAIRCARE FOR THE QUEENS WHO DO IT

MOMMY'S MANE

Bringing life into the world is magical—losing chunks of your hair afterward? Not so much. Postpartum shedding is real, but don't panic—your hair will bounce back with the right care. This section is all about strengthening those strands, soothing your scalp, and giving your hair the TLC it deserves after all your body has been through. Because mama, you're already a superhero—your hair just needs a little backup! Now, let's get into these recipes that'll have your mane thriving again!

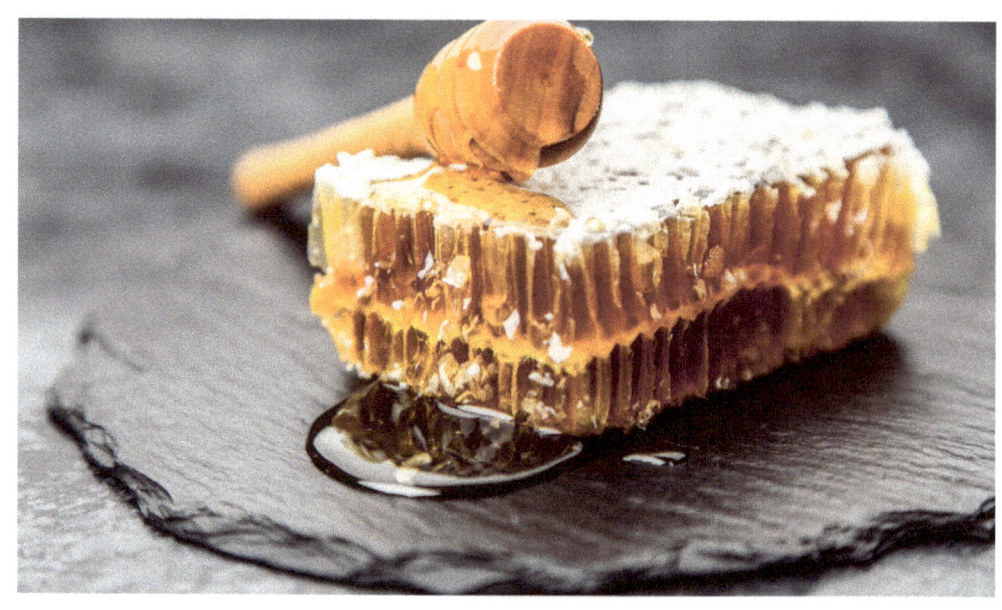

Mommy Magic Mask

POSTPARTUM RECOVERY BLEND

Ingredients

- 1 egg
- 1 tablespoon olive oil
- 1 tablespoon honey

Directions

1. Apply to damp hair
2. leave for 30 minutes
3. rinse thoroughly with cool water.

STRENGTHENING HAIR POST-PREGNANCY

Notes

Shelf Life: Use immediately; do not store.

Did you know?

Regular scalp massages can help stimulate blood circulation and promote hair growth by nourishing hair follicles.

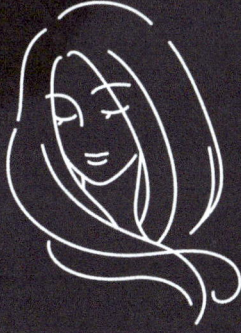

10

Chapter

CHEMICAL SERVICE.

CHEMICAL CONFIDENCE
THINK BEFORE YOU COMMIT

Color, relaxers, perms, and Brazilian treatments—oh my! These chemical services can transform your hair, but they also require real commitment. Whether you're smoothing things out with a Brazilian treatment, going bold with color, or keeping it sleek with a relaxer, the key to thriving hair is proper care before, during, and after the process. This section breaks down the do's and don'ts to keep your strands strong, balanced, and beautiful—because confidence starts with healthy hair!

Pro Tip:

Thinking of a major color change? Start small with highlights or a gloss treatment to test the waters.

CHEMICAL SERVICES:
THINK BEFORE YOU COMMIT

These can be game-changers, but they also require serious upkeep.

- Color Commitment is Real. If you're not ready to keep up with deep conditioning, regular trims, and hydration, step away from the dye bottle.
- Relaxers Need Caution. Over-processing can lead to thinning and breakage. Relaxers should always be done by a licensed professional.
- Protein & Moisture Balance. Chemical treatments strip the hair, so it's crucial to maintain protein-moisture balance.
- Stretch Your Touch-Ups. Avoid overlapping relaxer applications to prevent over-processing.
- Protect Your Scalp. Always ensure a protective base is applied before any chemical service to avoid burns and irritation.

11

Chapter

SHOPPING LIST

YOUR ULTIMATE STORE-BOUGHT HAIR CARE GUIDE:

What to Look For & What to Avoid?

Let's be real—sometimes life gets busy, and DIY just isn't in the cards. Whether you're always on the go, traveling, or simply prefer the convenience of store-bought products, knowing what to grab off the shelf can make all the difference. That's why I put together this guide—to help you shop smart and choose products that truly support your hair's health and goals.

No need to stress over brand names—this guide focuses on key ingredients to look for and those to avoid, so you can confidently pick products that align with your hair care needs. Whether you're maintaining a protective style, focusing on scalp health, or just looking to keep your strands moisturized and thriving, I've got you covered.

Let's dive in and break it all down!

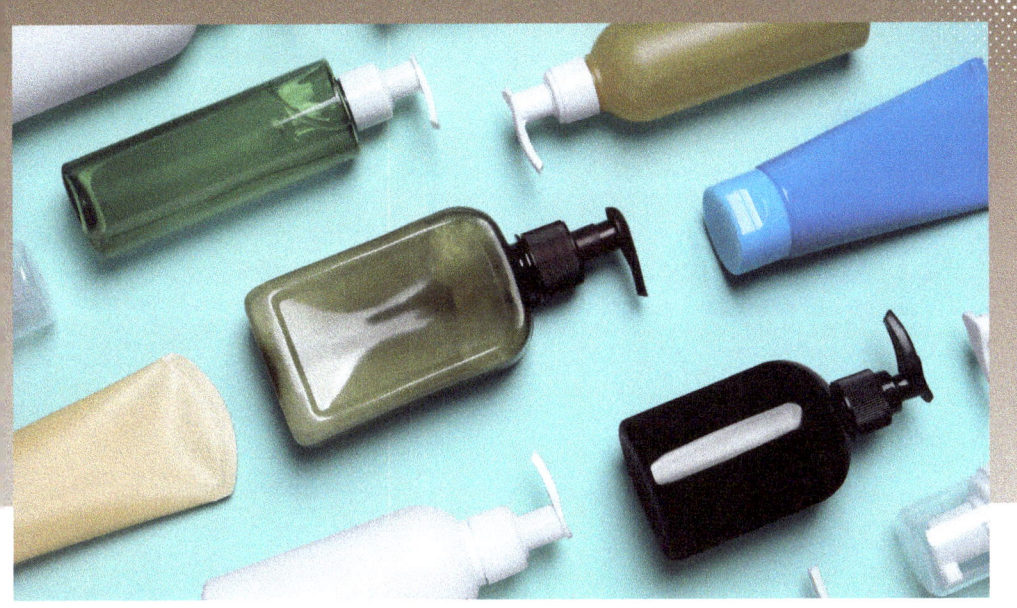

SHAMPOO & CLEANSERS:
CLEAN WITHOUT STRIPPING

Choosing the right shampoo is all about balance—
you want something that cleans your scalp without
leaving your hair feeling like straw.

What to Look For:

- Sulfate-free formulas – Gentle cleansers that won't strip your natural oils.
- Aloe vera, coconut milk, or oat protein – Hydration and soothing properties.
- Tea tree oil or apple cider vinegar – Helps with scalp buildup and dandruff control.
- pH-balanced formulas – Protects the scalp's natural barrier.

- Sulfates (SLS, SLES) – These strip too much moisture, leaving hair dry and prone to breakage.
- High alcohol content – Dries out the hair and scalp.
- Parabens and artificial fragrances – Can cause irritation over time.
- Heavy silicones – They coat the hair and can cause buildup over time.

Pro Tip:
Rotate between a moisturizing shampoo and a clarifying shampoo once a month to keep your scalp fresh and healthy.

CONDITIONERS & DEEP CONDITIONERS: MOISTURE IS KEY

A good conditioner should do more than just make your hair feel soft–it should strengthen, hydrate, and protect.

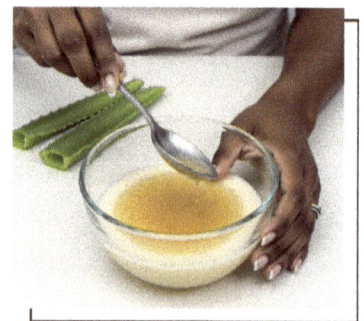

What to Look For:

- Water-based formulas – Look for water as the first ingredient for true hydration.
- Natural oils like avocado, jojoba, or olive oil – For lasting moisture.
- Protein blends like hydrolyzed keratin or silk protein – Helps strengthen weak strands.
- Ingredients like marshmallow root or slippery elm – Adds slip for easier detangling.

What to Avoid:

- Products with excessive silicones – These can provide temporary smoothness but lead to buildup.
- Parabens and phthalates – Linked to scalp irritation.
- Heavy waxes and petrolatum – These can clog the hair and scalp, leading to dryness underneath.

Pro Tip:
Deep condition weekly for intense hydration and strength—your hair will thank you.

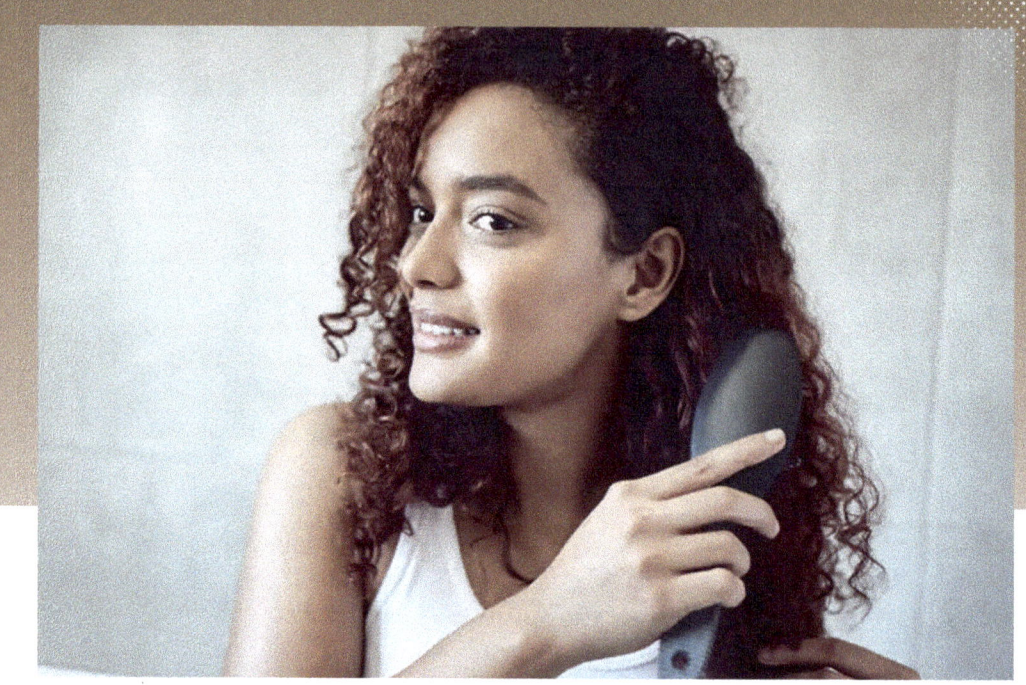

LEAVE-IN CONDITIONERS:
DAILY MOISTURE MATTERS

The right leave-in conditioner should keep your hair hydrated, soft, and manageable without weighing it down.

What to Look For:

- Aloe vera or rose water – Lightweight hydration that won't cause buildup.
- Humectants like glycerin or panthenol – Pulls moisture into the hair.
- Lightweight oils like argan or grapeseed – Helps seal in moisture without a greasy feel.
- Protein if needed – Great for damaged hair that needs strength.

- Products with mineral oil – It coats the hair rather than nourishing it.
- Drying alcohols (ethanol, isopropyl alcohol) – These can leave your hair brittle.
- Heavy butter-based formulas – Better suited for styling, not as a leave-in.

Pro Tip:

Choose a creamy leave-in for thick, curly hair, and a lightweight spray for finer textures.

OILS & MOISTURIZERS:
SEAL THE DEAL

Locking in moisture is crucial, and the right oils and moisturizers can make all the difference.

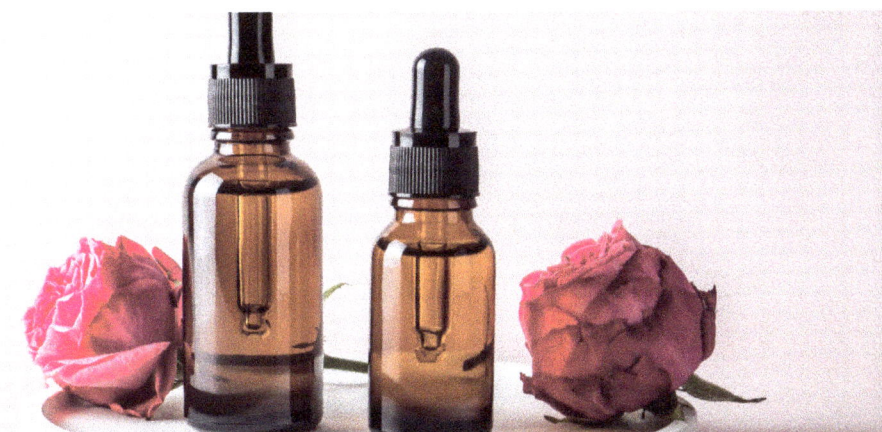

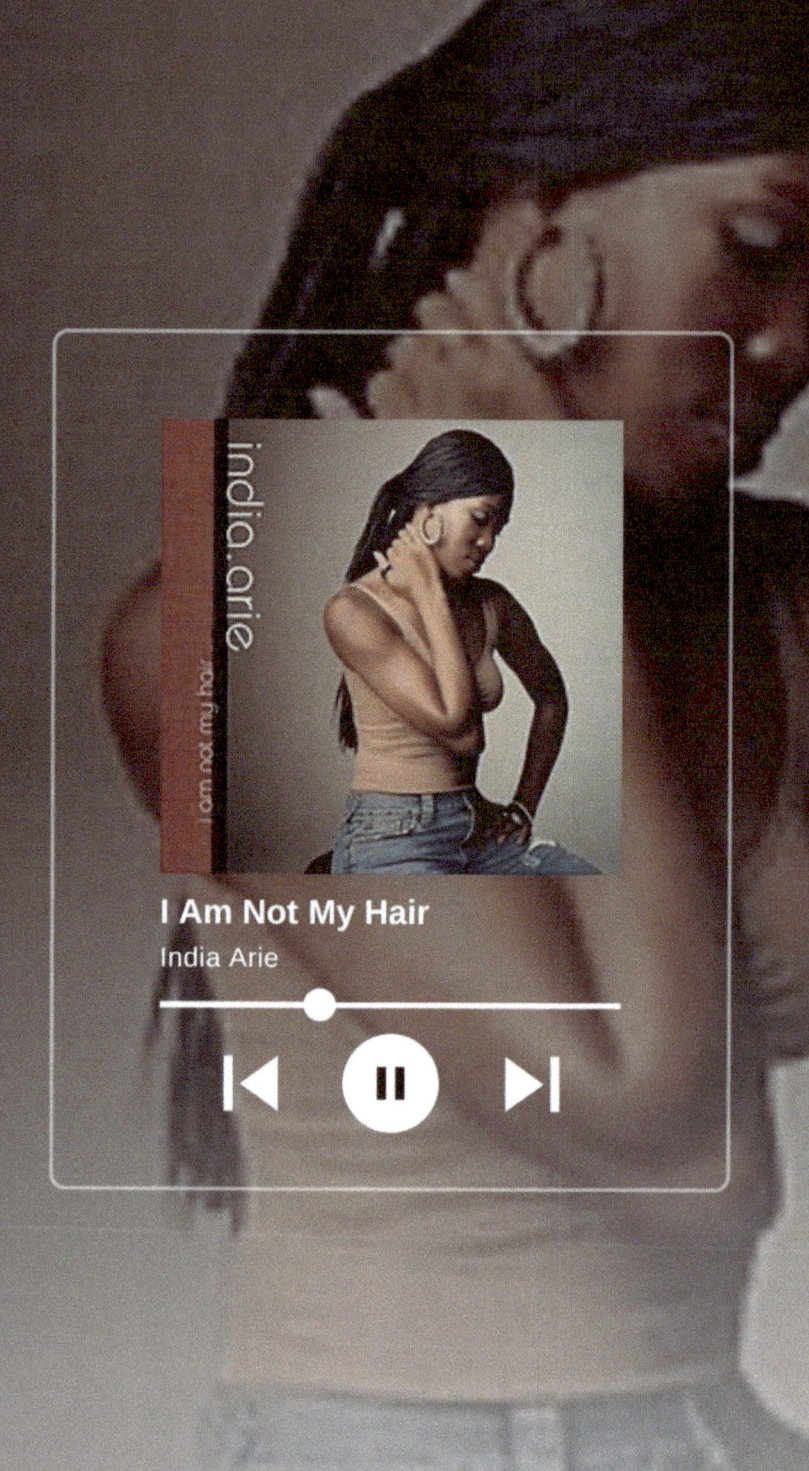

I Am Not My Hair
India Arie

What to Look For:

- Cold-pressed, natural oils such as:
- Jojoba oil – Mimics natural scalp oils.
- Castor oil – Promotes hair growth and thickness.
- Avocado oil – Deeply nourishes dry hair.
- Sweet almond oil – Lightweight and perfect for fine strands.
- Cream-based moisturizers – Look for aloe vera or shea butter for lasting hydration.

What to Avoid:

- Mineral oil and petroleum – They block moisture from penetrating the hair shaft.
- Synthetic fragrance oils – These can lead to scalp irritation.

Pro Tip:
Always apply oils on damp hair to seal in moisture and avoid unnecessary dryness.

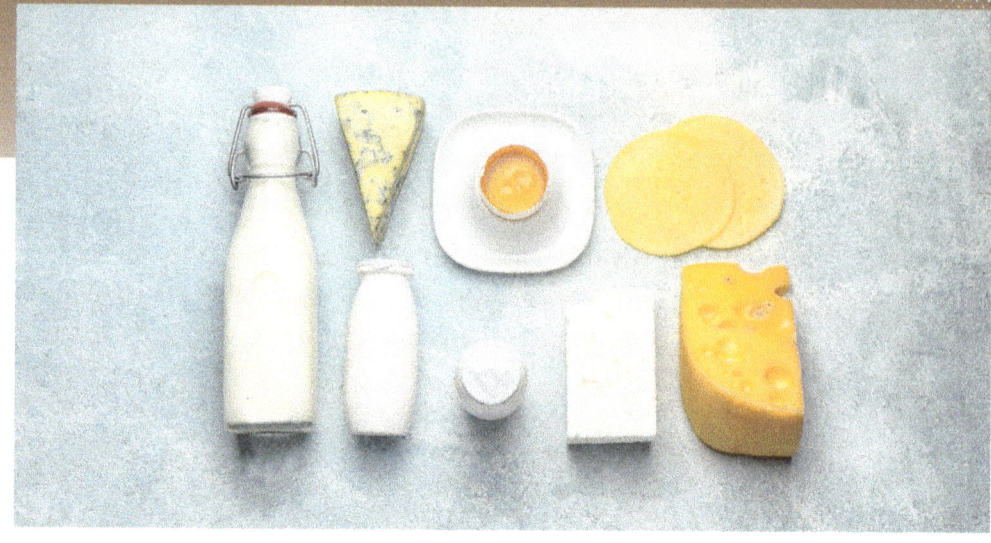

STYLING PRODUCTS:
DEFINE WITHOUT DAMAGE

Whether you're rocking a twist-out, wash-and-go, or slick-back, the right styling product can make or break your look.

What to Look For:

- Flaxseed or aloe vera-based gels – Provides hold without stiffness.
- Butters like mango or shea – Perfect for twist-outs and braid-outs.
- Flexible hold formulas – Keeps hair soft yet defined.

What to Avoid:

- Alcohol-heavy gels – Can dry out curls and leave flakes.
- Sticky wax-based products – Can cause buildup and clogged follicles.

Pro Tip:
Layer your styling products with a leave-in conditioner first to avoid crunchiness.

SCALP TREATMENTS:
NOURISH FROM THE ROOT

A healthy scalp is the foundation of healthy hair. Treat it well!

What to Look For:

- Tea tree or peppermint oil – Great for stimulating and clarifying the scalp.
- Witch hazel or aloe vera – Soothes itchiness and irritation.
- Scalp scrubs with gentle exfoliants – Removes buildup without irritation.

What to Avoid:

- Products with artificial dyes and fragrance – Can irritate sensitive scalps.
- Heavy oils applied directly to the scalp – Can clog hair follicles if overused.

Pro Tip:
Massage your scalp daily for 5 minutes to encourage blood flow and hair growth.

FOR THE FELLAS:
MEN'S GROOMING ESSENTIALS

A healthy scalp is the foundation of healthy hair. Treat it well!

What to Look For:

- Beard oils with jojoba or argan oil – Helps keep facial hair soft and nourished.
- Sulfate-free shampoos – Cleanses hair without stripping.
- Lightweight leave-ins – Keeps hair hydrated without a greasy feel.

What to Avoid:

- Heavy, waxy products – Can clog pores and lead to breakouts.
- Fragrance-heavy products – Can cause irritation.

Pro Tip: Keep your beard hydrated daily with a light oil to avoid flakiness and itchiness.

FINAL THOUGHTS:

Smarter Shopping for Healthier Hair

Now that you know what to look for and what to avoid, shopping for hair care just got a whole lot easier. Take your time, read those labels, and always choose products that align with your hair's needs.

Because healthy hair starts with smart choices— whether DIY or store-bought!

Did you know?

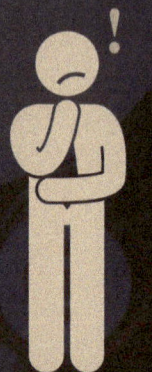

Natural ingredients like aloe vera, avocado, and honey can deeply nourish textured hair and promote moisture retention.

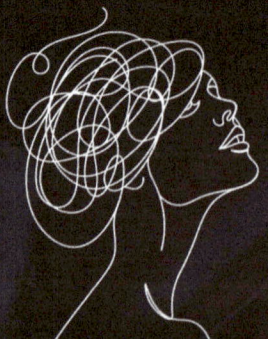

12

Chapter

UGH, NOTHING IS WORKING

EXPLORING OTHER OPTIONS:
WHAT ELSE IS OUT THERE?

While I'm all about DIY and natural hair care, I know that sometimes you might be looking for additional solutions—especially when dealing with significant hair loss or stubborn growth challenges. If you've tried everything and your hair just isn't cooperating, there are other options out there that people explore, including:

Minoxidil (a.k.a. "that popular hair regrowth solution")

Minoxidil is an FDA-approved topical treatment that some people use to encourage hair regrowth. It's widely available, but results can vary, and it requires consistent use. Before diving in, it's always best to have a chat with your healthcare provider to see if it's right for you.

Oral Supplements

From biotin to collagen, supplements claim to support hair growth from the inside out. While some swear by them, others find that balanced nutrition does the trick. Just remember—more isn't always better, and it's always wise to check with your doctor before starting any supplement routine.

Hair Transplants

When hair loss is more advanced, some people consider professional solutions like hair transplants. This involves moving hair follicles from one part of your scalp to another. It's a commitment, both financially and physically, so make sure to do thorough research and consult with a specialist if this is something you're curious about.

At the end of the day, your hair journey is personal, and there's no one-size-fits-all solution. Whether you choose a DIY route, explore medical treatments, or a mix of both, what matters most is making informed choices that work for you. And remember—there's no shame in seeking professional help if you need it!

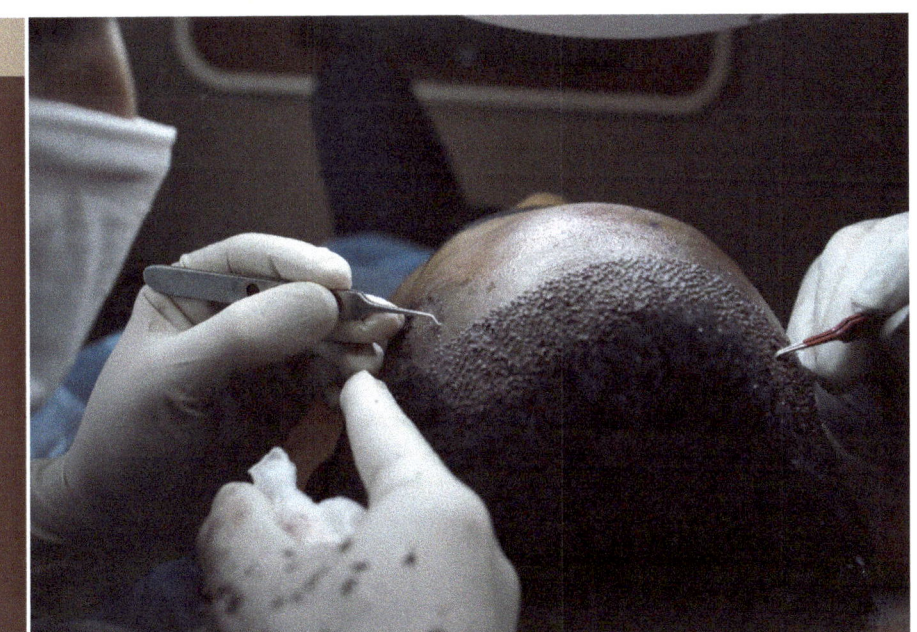

▶ When to Seek Professional Help for Your Hair Concerns

Sometimes, no matter how much love and care you give your hair, things just don't seem to improve. If you're experiencing persistent hair loss, excessive shedding, or scalp issues that don't respond to at-home treatments, it might be time to call in the pros.

A dermatologist or trichologist (a hair and scalp specialist) can provide a thorough analysis and help identify underlying issues—whether it's hormonal imbalances, scalp conditions, or nutritional deficiencies that could be impacting your hair's health.

Signs It Might Be Time to See a Professional:

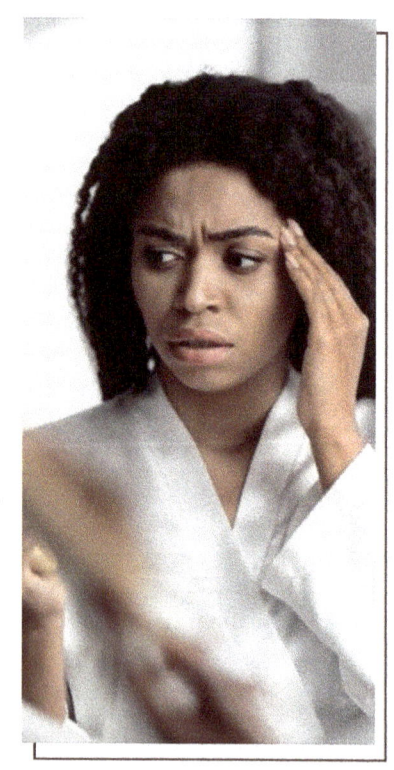

- Sudden or excessive hair shedding that doesn't improve with lifestyle changes.
- Itchy, flaky, or irritated scalp that persists despite regular care.
- Thinning hair or bald patches appearing unexpectedly.
- Breakage that worsens over time, even with protective measures.
- Changes in hair texture that seem unusual or concerning.

Seeking professional advice doesn't mean you've failed—it means you're taking your hair health seriously and want to get to the root (literally) of the issue. A dermatologist or trichologist can recommend medical treatments, lifestyle changes, or even guide you on how to adjust your hair care routine to better suit your needs.

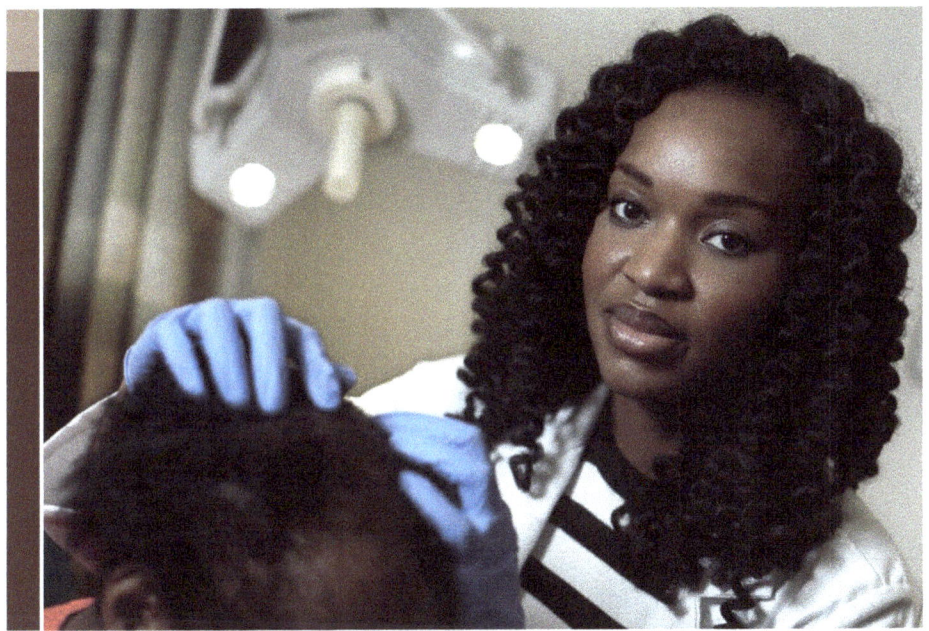

Pro Tip:
Keep a hair journal (hint, hint!) to track your progress, symptoms, and routines. This can be helpful when discussing your concerns with a professional.

At the end of the day, your hair deserves the best care possible—whether that means DIY treatments, store-bought solutions, or a little extra help from the experts.

When to Seek Professional Help for Your Hair Concerns

Sometimes, no matter how much love and care you give your hair, things just don't seem to improve. If you're experiencing persistent hair loss, excessive shedding, or scalp issues that don't respond to at-home treatments, it might be time to call in the pros.

A dermatologist or trichologist (a hair and scalp specialist) can provide a thorough analysis and help identify underlying issues—whether it's hormonal imbalances, scalp conditions, or nutritional deficiencies that could be impacting your hair's health.

IF IT DOESN'T NOURISH YOUR SOUL OR YOUR **HAIR**, LET IT GO.

Did you know?

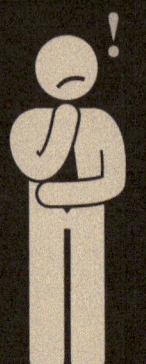

Your hair's porosity level (low, normal, or high) determines how well it absorbs and retains moisture, which affects product effectiveness.

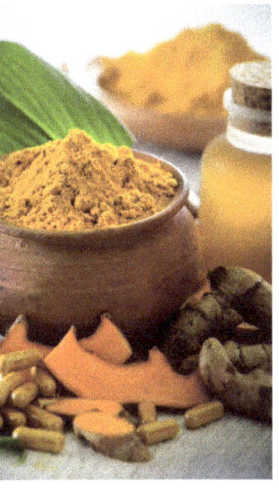

Herbs & Powders for DIY Treatments

- Amla powder (strengthens hair and scalp)
- Hibiscus powder (adds shine and promotes growth)
- Henna powder (natural hair strengthening)
- Fenugreek powder (moisture and growth)
- Brahmi powder (reduces hair fall)

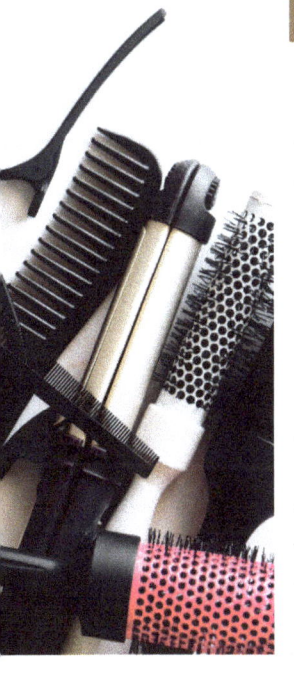

Styling Products & Tools

- Satin or silk scarf/bonnet (reduces breakage)
- Spray bottle (for refreshing curls)
- Wide-tooth comb (gentle detangling)
- Microfiber towel or t-shirt (reduces frizz)
- Edge control gel (for sleek styles)
- Heat protectant spray (for styling)
- Flexible rods or perm rods (for heatless curls)
- Hair clips or sectioning tools
- Scalp massager (stimulates growth)

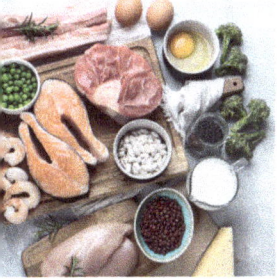

Protein & Strengthening Ingredients

- Hydrolyzed keratin (strengthens strands)
- Silk protein (smooths and strengthens)
- Collagen powder (for elasticity)

DIY Moisturizing Ingredients

- Vegetable glycerin (moisture retention)
- Marshmallow root (detangling benefits)
- Slippery elm (softens hair and reduces breakage)

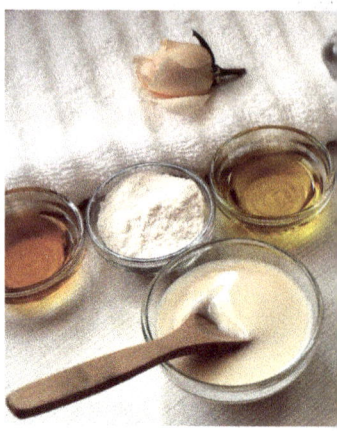

Shampoo & Cleansing Must-Haves

- African black soap (gentle cleansing)
- Rhassoul clay (natural cleanser)
- Bentonite clay (deep scalp detox)

Protective Style Essentials

- Satin-lined caps (for braids and wigs)
- Lightweight leave-in conditioners
- Braid spray (for scalp hydration)
- Edge scarf (to lay those edges)
- Stocking caps (for wig protection)

Hydration Boosters

- Distilled water (pure base for DIY sprays)
- Cucumber juice (scalp refreshment)
- Aloe vera gel (hydration and healing)

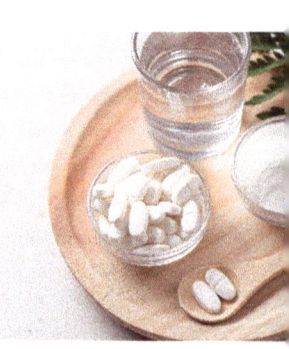

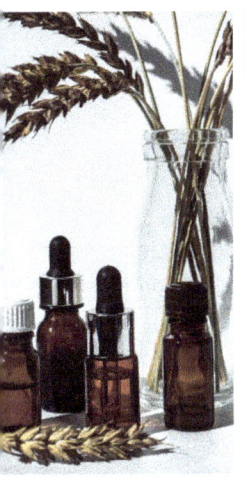

Quick Add-On Essentials

- Measuring spoons (for accurate DIY mixing)
- Mixing bowls (for DIY concoctions)
- Applicator bottles (for scalp treatments)
- Plastic caps (for deep conditioning treatments)
- Wooden spoon (avoid metal when mixing clays)

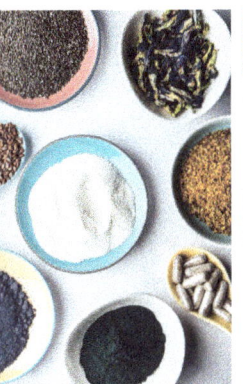

Healthy Hair from the Inside Out (Supplements)

- Biotin supplements
- Omega-3 fatty acids
- Collagen peptides
- MSM powder (for growth support)
- Multivitamins (support overall hair health)

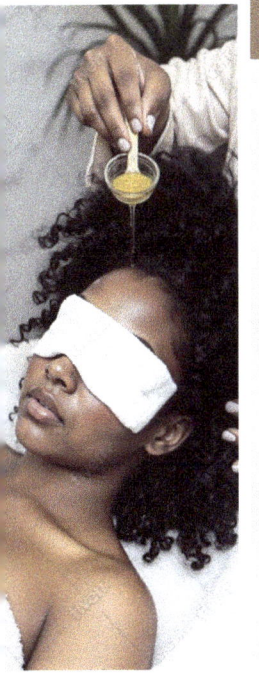

Pro Tips for Shopping Success:

- Check your pantry first! You might already have some of these ingredients at home.
- Quality over quantity. Invest in organic, cold-pressed, and unrefined ingredients for the best results.
- DIY storage matters. Glass jars and dark bottles help keep your homemade products fresh longer.
- Start small. Buy in small quantities to test what works best for your hair before stocking up.

When your hair is happy, you're happy! Stock up, experiment, and find what works best for YOUR crown.

Did you know?

Over-washing your hair can strip away natural oils that keep it healthy, leading to dryness and breakage.

13

Chapter

ALOPECIA

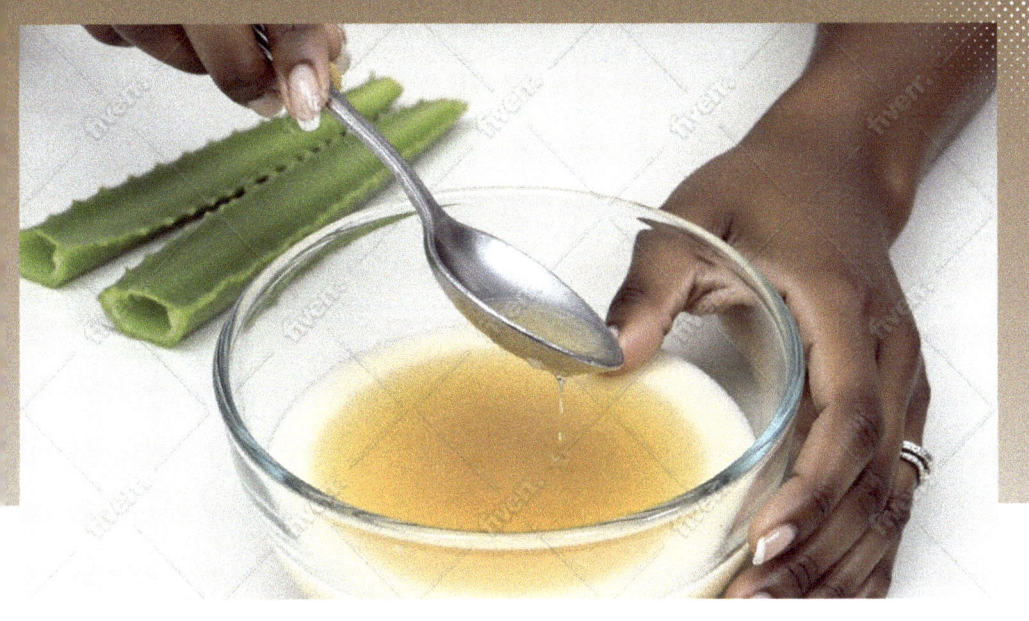

ALOPECIA AREATA:
UNDERSTANDING, CARING, AND THRIVING

Hair loss can be an emotional journey, and if you're dealing with Alopecia Areata, know that you're not alone. It's a condition that affects many people, and while it can be challenging, there are ways to care for your hair and scalp that nurture both your strands and your confidence.

Alopecia Areata is an autoimmune condition that can cause sudden hair loss in small, round patches on the scalp and other areas of the body. It can come and go unexpectedly, and while it doesn't cause physical pain, the emotional impact can be real. The good news? With the right knowledge, care, and patience, you can support your hair's health and feel empowered on your journey.

Listening to Your Hair

Pay attention to how your hair and scalp feel. If your hair feels greasy, heavy, or your scalp is itchy, it might be time for a wash. Conversely, if your hair feels dry or brittle, consider spacing out your washes and incorporating moisturizing treatments.

Alternative Cleansing Methods:

Co-Washing: Using a conditioner to wash your hair can be a gentler alternative, helping to maintain moisture while still cleansing the scalp.

Dry Shampoo: On days when you want to skip a full wash, a dry shampoo can help absorb excess oil and keep your hair looking fresh.

> **"**
> Remember, there's no one-size-fits-all answer. It's about finding a routine that keeps your hair healthy and makes you feel your best.
> **"**

Life is short.
Make each
hair flip
fabulous!

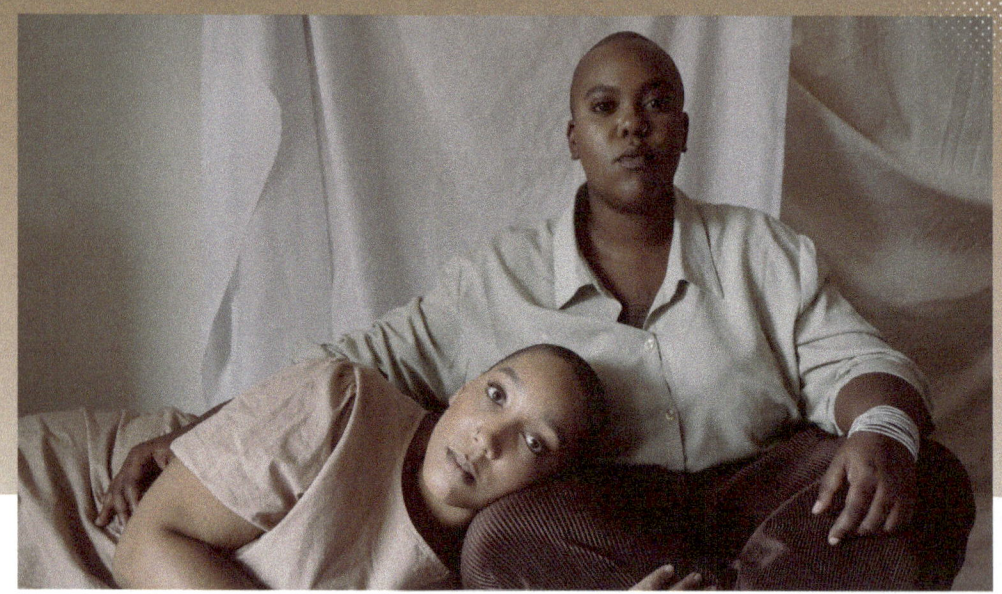

ALOPECIA AREATA: THE DOS & DON'TS

Let's get into some key things to do (and avoid) to best support your hair and scalp.

DO:

☐ Consult a Professional
A licensed dermatologist or trichologist can provide personalized advice, recommend treatments, and guide you through options that best suit your condition.

☐ Be Gentle with Your Hair
Opt for low-manipulation styles and gentle detangling methods to avoid unnecessary tension.

☐ Nourish from Within
Eating a balanced diet rich in iron, zinc, vitamin D, and biotin can help support hair regrowth from the inside out.

☐ Massage Your Scalp
Regular, gentle scalp massages with lightweight oils can improve circulation and encourage growth.

☐ Protect Your Hair
Sleep with a satin or silk scarf to reduce friction and keep your strands protected.

☐ Stay Positive and Patient
Hair regrowth takes time, but with consistent care and a holistic approach, progress is possible.

DON'T:

☐ Ignore the Signs
If you're noticing sudden or excessive hair loss, seek professional help sooner rather than later.

☐ Overmanipulate Your Hair
Avoid tight ponytails, braids, or styles that put stress on thinning areas.

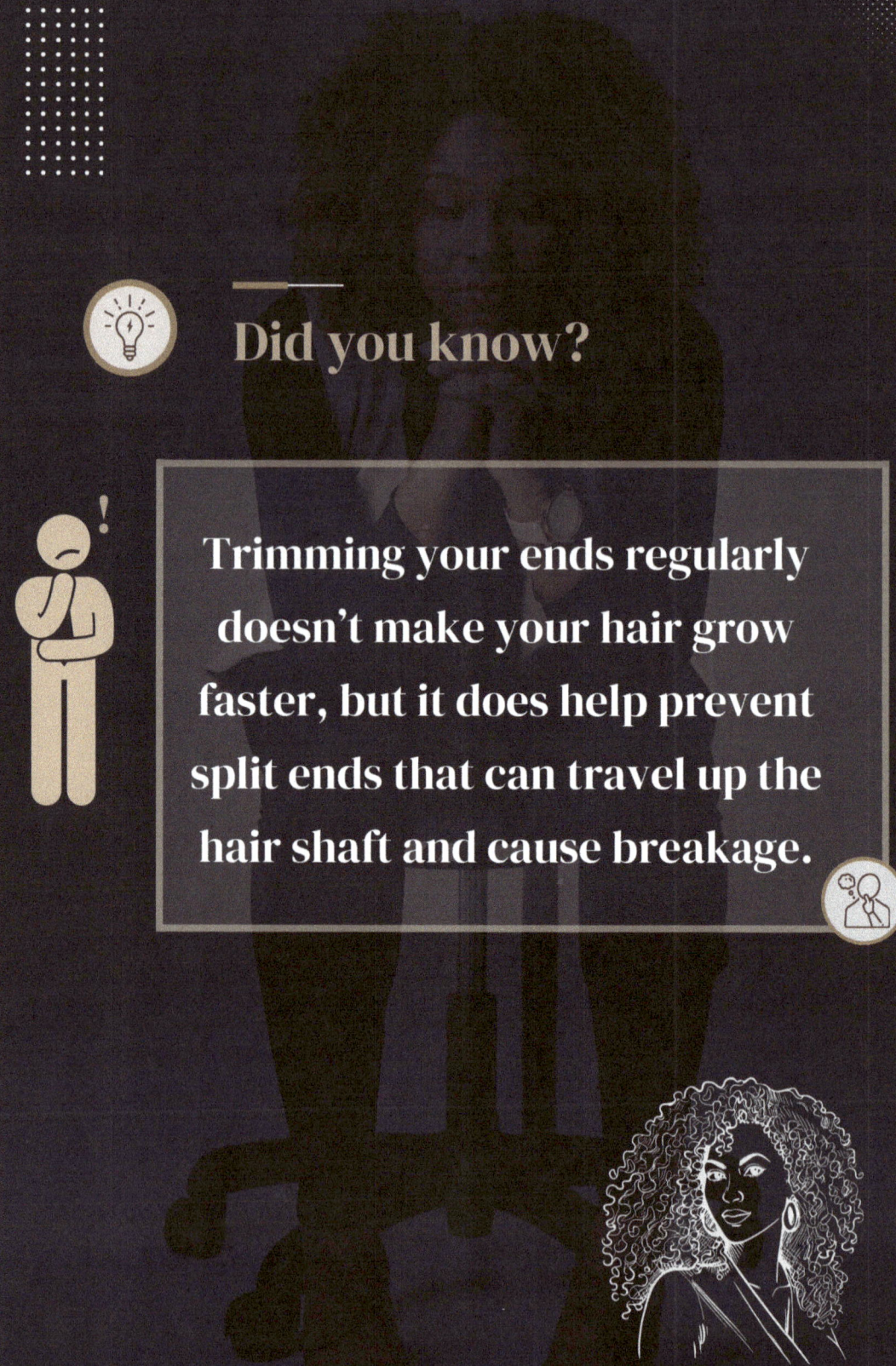

Did you know?

Trimming your ends regularly doesn't make your hair grow faster, but it does help prevent split ends that can travel up the hair shaft and cause breakage.

DIY Remedies for Alopecia Areata

Here are some gentle, effective DIY treatments that can help nourish the scalp and encourage healthy regrowth.

Scalp-Stimulating Hair Growth Oil

Nourish and strengthen hair follicles with this lightweight, nutrient-rich blend.

Ingredients:

- 2 tbsp castor oil (stimulates hair growth)
- 1 tbsp black seed oil (anti-inflammatory benefits)
- 1 tbsp argan oil (moisturizing and strengthening)
- 5 drops rosemary essential oil (proven to encourage regrowth)
- 3 drops peppermint essential oil (increases circulation)

Instructions:

1. Mix all ingredients in a small glass dropper bottle.
2. Apply 2-3 drops to affected areas and gently massage for 5 minutes.
3. Use 3-4 times a week for best results.

> **Pro Tip:** Try using a scalp massager to enhance absorption and blood flow.

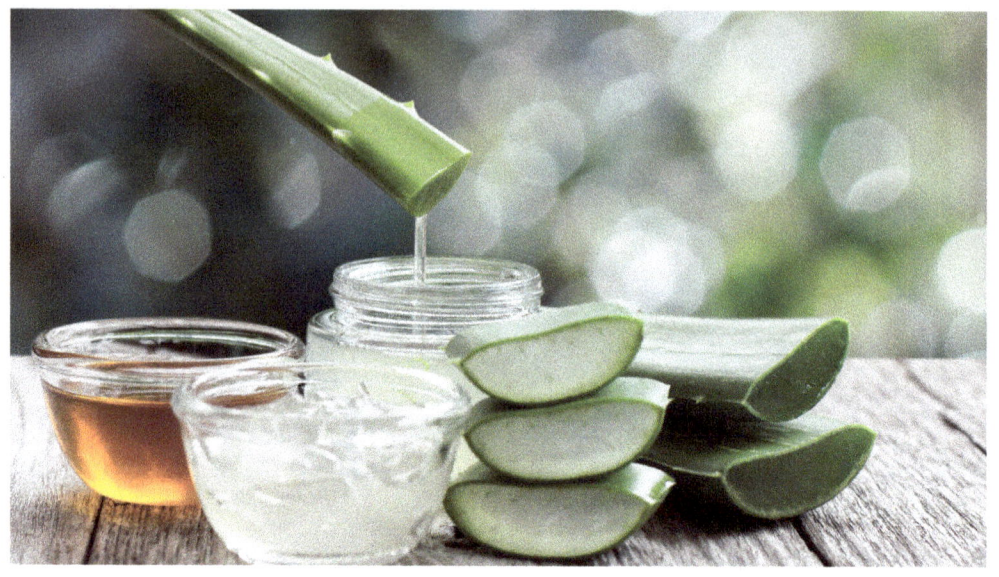

Aloe Vera & Onion Juice Scalp Treatment

Onion juice contains sulfur, which helps with follicle stimulation, while aloe vera soothes and hydrates the scalp.

Ingredients

- 2 tbsp aloe vera gel (hydrates and soothes)
- 1 tbsp onion juice (stimulates follicles)
- 1 tsp honey (locks in moisture and reduces irritation)

Instructions:

- Blend ingredients into a smooth mixture.
- Apply directly to the scalp, focusing on thinning areas.
- Let sit for 30 minutes, then rinse with lukewarm water and a gentle shampoo.

Pro Tip:

Use once a week to reduce inflammation and support hair regrowth.

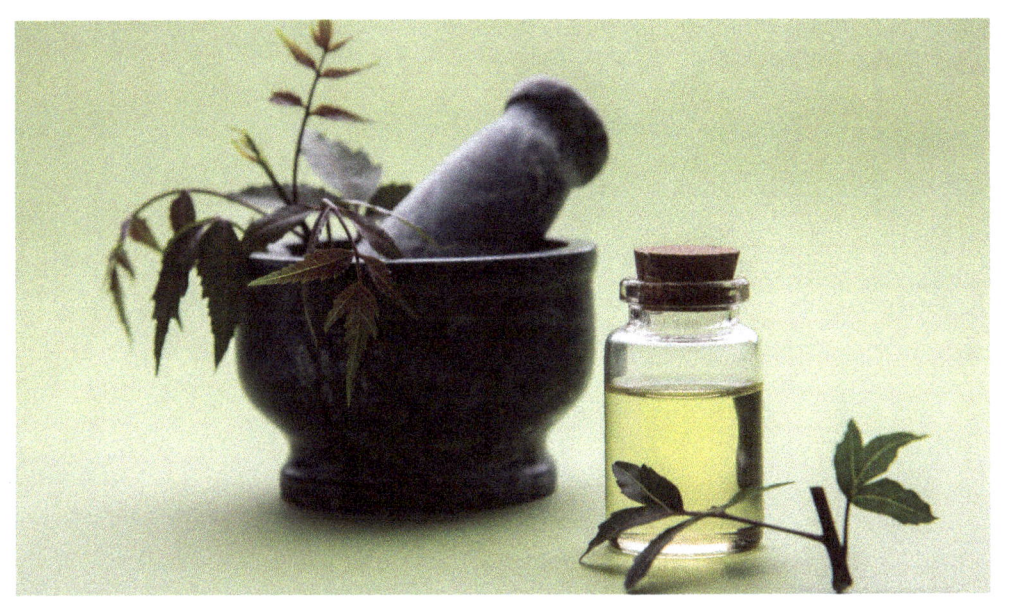

Ayurvedic Hair Mask for Strengthening

This mask is packed with antioxidants to promote scalp health and nourish thinning areas.

Ingredients

- 2 tbsp amla powder (rich in vitamin C and antioxidants)
- 1 tbsp fenugreek powder (strengthens and thickens hair)
- 1 tbsp hibiscus powder (supports scalp health)
- 1/2 cup coconut milk (deep hydration and nourishment)

Instructions:

- Mix all ingredients into a paste.
- Apply evenly to the scalp and hair, focusing on affected areas.
- Leave on for 30-45 minutes before rinsing with warm water.

Pro Tip:

Use every two weeks for best results.

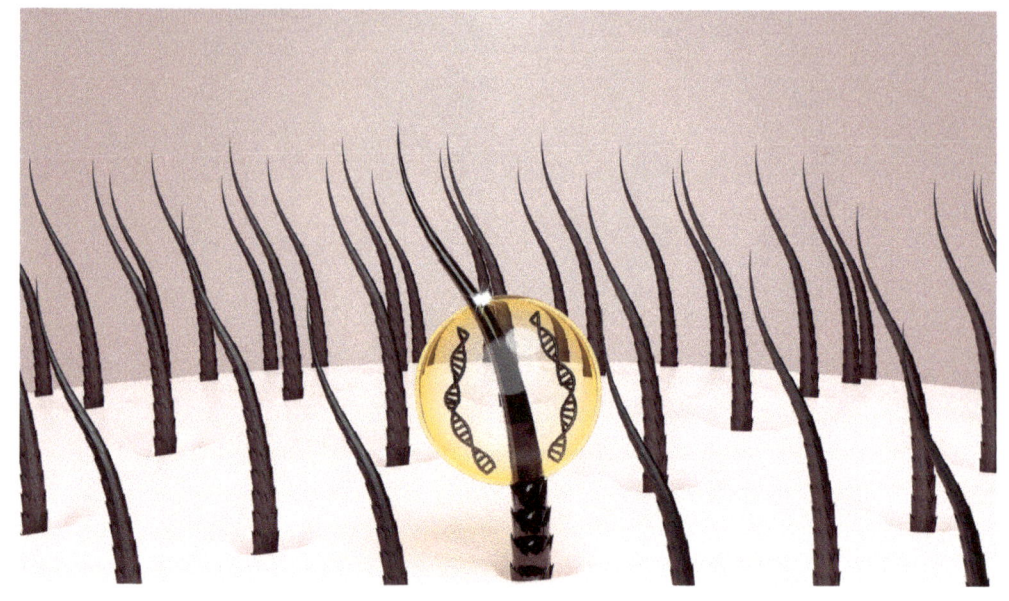

Green Tea Rinse for Hair Follicle Support

Green tea contains antioxidants that fight inflammation and may help reactivate hair follicles.

Ingredients

- 2 green tea bags
- 1 cup hot water
- 1 tbsp apple cider vinegar (balances scalp pH)

Instructions:

- Steep the green tea bags in hot water for 15 minutes, then cool.
- Add apple cider vinegar and stir well.
- Pour over the scalp after shampooing and massage gently.
- Rinse after 5-10 minutes.

Pro Tip:
Use after each wash day to boost scalp health.

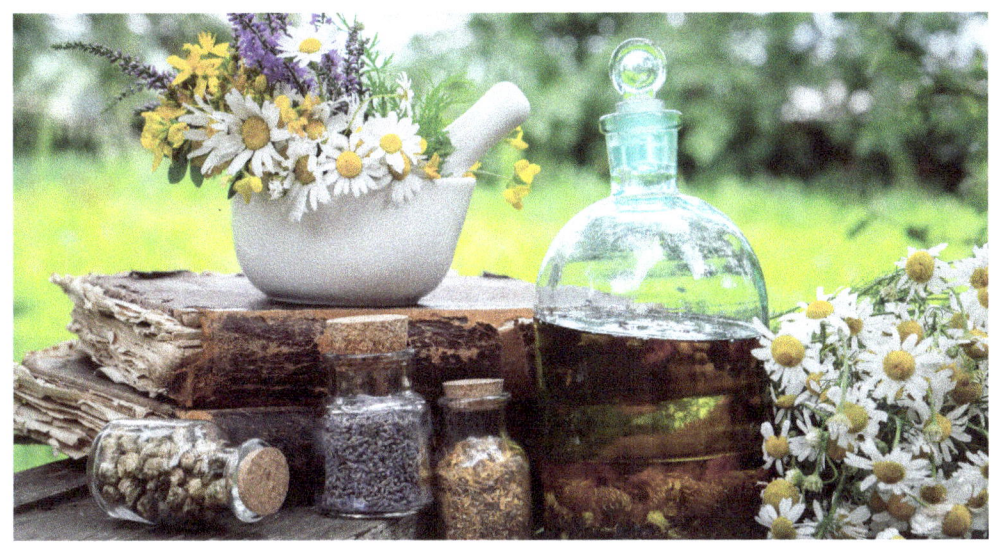

Chebe Crown Elixir

Length-Retaining Hair Mask

Ingredients

- 2 tablespoons Chebe powder
- 2 tablespoons castor oil (for strength) or coconut oil (for moisture)
- 2 tablespoons shea butter (optional for extra hydration)
- 1/4 cup warm water or aloe vera juice (adjust for desired consistency)

Instructions:

- Mix all ingredients in a bowl until a smooth, thick paste forms.
- Section your hair, focusing on the mid-lengths and ends (avoid direct scalp application).
- Apply generously, then braid or twist your hair for better absorption.
- Leave on for 1-2 hours (or overnight for intense hydration).
- Rinse thoroughly with lukewarm water and follow with a gentle shampoo and conditioner.

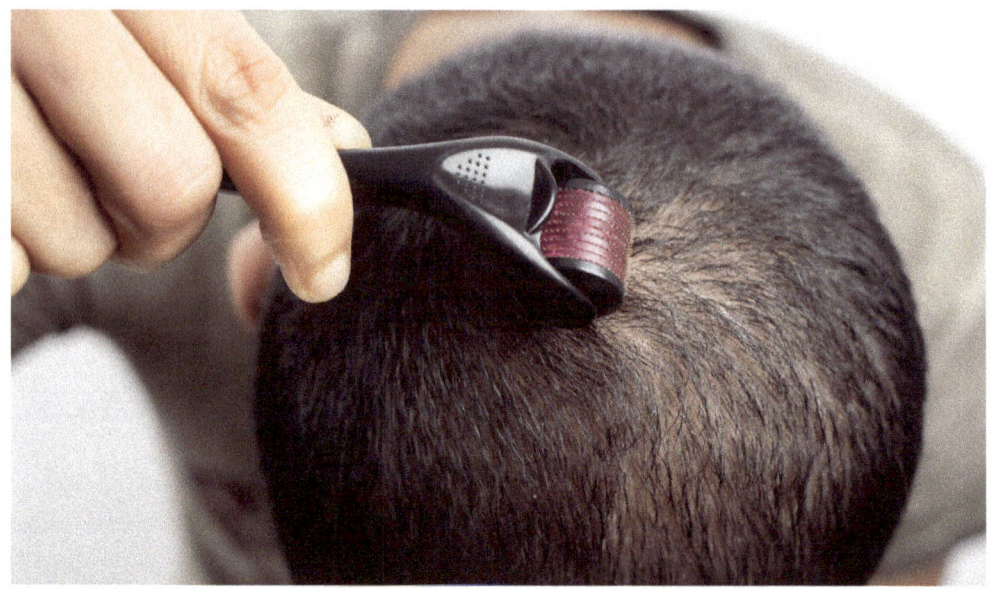

Scalp Soothing Mask for Irritation Relief

Perfect for calming inflammation and adding essential moisture to affected areas.

Ingredients

- 2 tbsp aloe vera gel (soothes and hydrates)
- 1 tbsp oatmeal (calms irritation)
- 1 tsp coconut oil (locks in moisture)

Instructions:

- Blend ingredients into a smooth paste.
- Apply directly to the scalp, concentrating on sensitive areas.
- Leave for 20 minutes and rinse thoroughly.

Pro Tip:

Use weekly to maintain scalp comfort and hydration.

FINAL THOUGHTS ON ALOPECIA CARE

Caring for hair affected by alopecia takes patience, consistency, and a lot of love. Remember, healthy hair starts with a healthy scalp and the right mindset. Don't be discouraged–take it one day at a time, and celebrate every win along the way.

If hair regrowth feels slow, focus on nurturing what you have, trying different styles that make you feel beautiful, and seeking professional advice when needed.

Your hair is your crown–wear it with confidence, no matter what stage you're in.

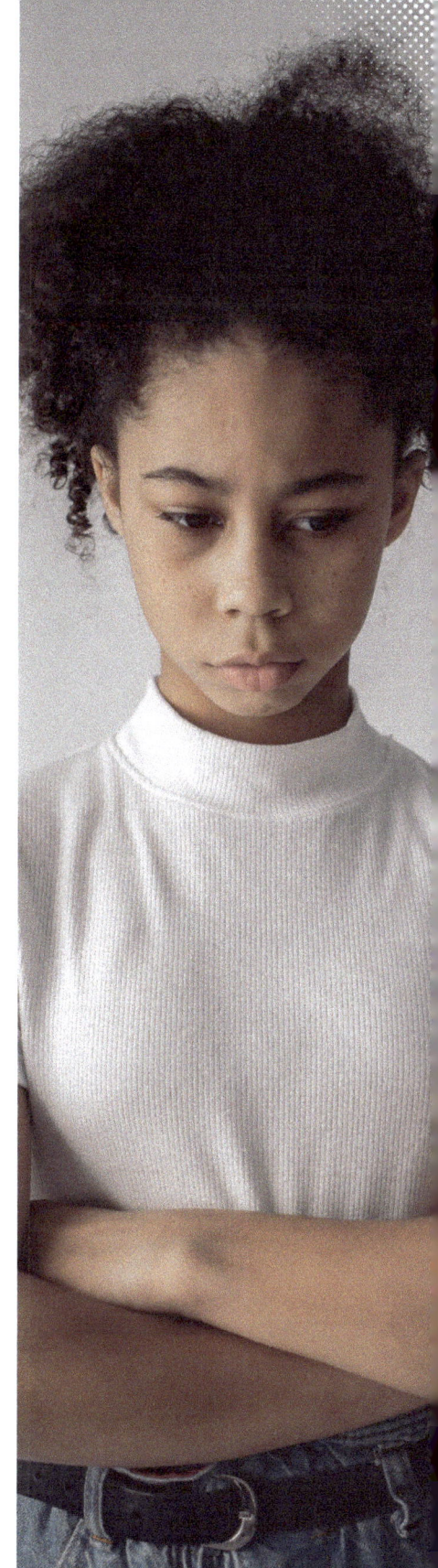

14

Chapter

FINDING YOUR
CROWNS KEEPER

FROM HORROR STORIES TO HAIR GLORY: FINDING YOUR CROWN'S KEEPER

We've all heard the tales—appointments that start late, stylists who double-book, and salons where professionalism is as scarce as a comb in a bald man's bathroom. But here's the tea: it's time to raise our standards and reclaim our time (and edges). Your hair is your crown, and it deserves a stylist who treats it—and you—with the utmost respect.

THE NEW STANDARD:
Professionalism in Black Hair Salons

It's become all too common to expect subpar service in some Black hair salons. But let's be clear: professionalism should be the rule, not the exception. Punctuality, cleanliness, and respect are non-negotiables. As clients, we must demand better and not settle for the bare minimum just to get our hair laid.

Red Flags to Watch Out For

Before you sit in that chair, keep an eye out for these warning signs:

Lack of Consultation:

If a stylist doesn't ask about your hair history or desired outcome, consider it a red flag. A thorough consultation is crucial for achieving the best results.

Dirty or Disorganized Space:

A clean salon reflects a stylist's professionalism. If the salon is unkempt, it might be best to look elsewhere.

Unfriendly Staff:

You should feel welcomed and comfortable. Rude or dismissive behavior is unacceptable.

GREEN LIGHTS:
SIGNS OF A GREAT STYLIST

Look for these positive indicators:

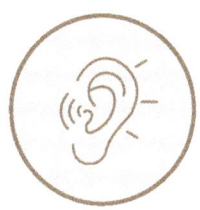

Active Listening:
A stylist who listens to your preferences and asks questions about your hair type and desired style is a keeper.

Ongoing Education:
Stylists who stay updated on the latest techniques and trends demonstrate a commitment to their craft.

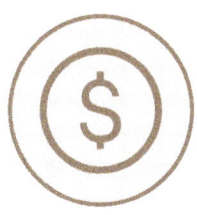

Transparent Pricing:
Clear communication about costs upfront helps build trust and ensures there are no surprises.

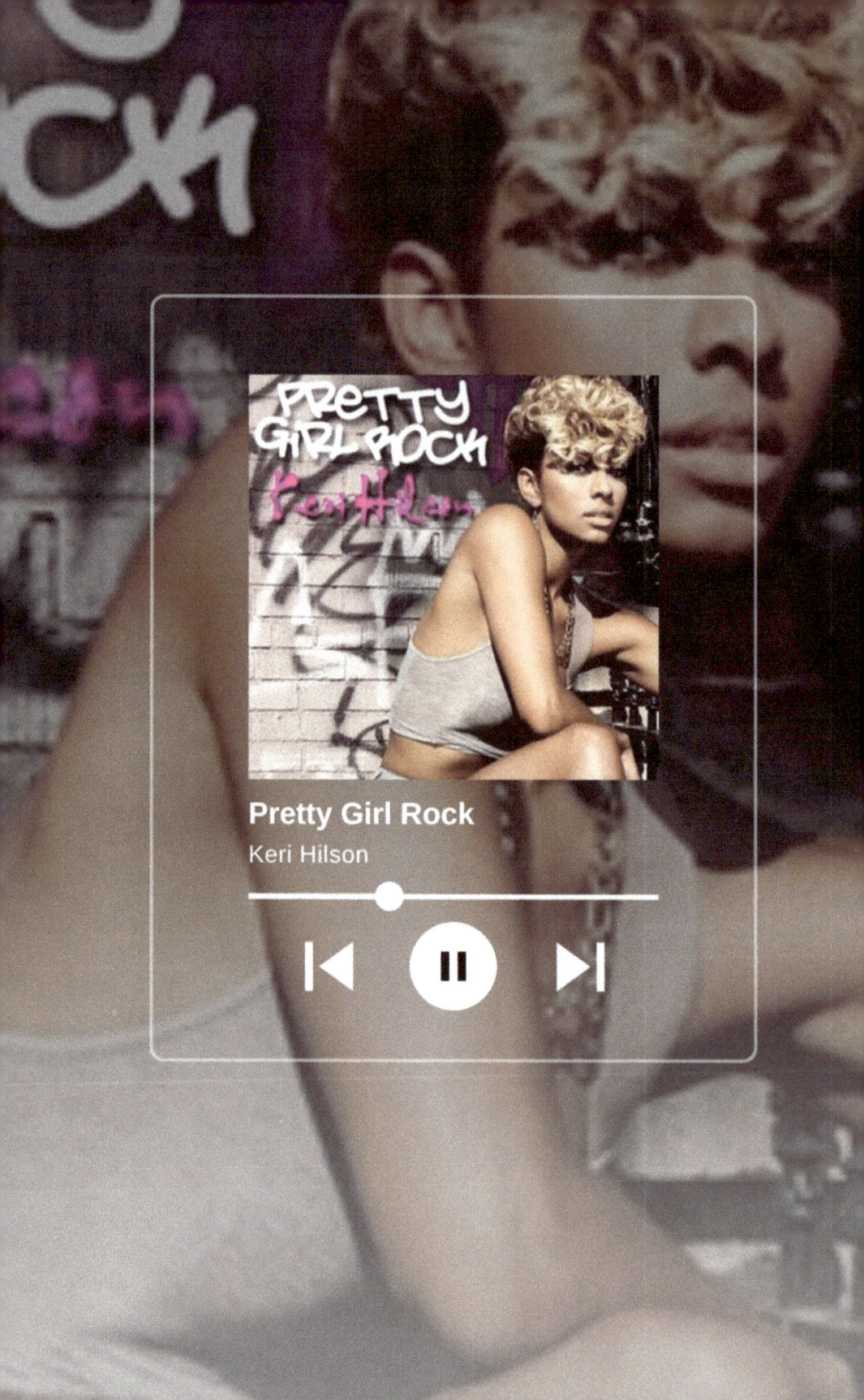

Pretty Girl Rock

Keri Hilson

DOING YOUR HOMEWORK:
RESEARCH AND REVIEWS

In this digital age, there's no excuse for not doing your research. Check online reviews, ask for recommendations, and don't hesitate to consult multiple stylists before making your decision. Remember, you're not just paying for a service; you're investing in your hair's health and your peace of mind.

CONCLUSION

Your hair journey is personal, and finding the right stylist is a crucial part of that path. By setting high standards and refusing to accept less, you not only ensure better service for yourself but also elevate the industry as a whole. So, hold your head high, do your research, and find that stylist who will make your hair—and your spirit—shine.

Remember, queens:
your crown deserves nothing less than the best.

THE FIXER-UPPER CREW:
VITAMINS FOR SPECIFIC HAIR PROBLEMS

▶ **Hair Shedding?**
Iron, Vitamin D, and Biotin can help keep your strands where they belong—on your head, not your brush.

▶ **Dry, Brittle Hair?**
Omega-3s, Vitamin E, and Collagen are your hydration heroes.

▶ **Slow Growth?**
Biotin, Vitamin D, and Zinc can help wake up your follicles and get them working again.

▶ **Thinning Edges?**
Vitamin B12 and Iron keep your scalp nourished and your hairline thriving.

Final Word: Don't Play Yourself

Listen, sis. Vitamins aren't a quick fix—you won't wake up tomorrow with Rapunzel inches, but consistent intake will help your hair, skin, and overall health glow up over time. Just pair these with a healthy diet and plenty of water, and you'll be unstoppable.

Now go ahead and add these to your daily routine —your hair will thank you later!

15

Chapter

SHOPPING LIST

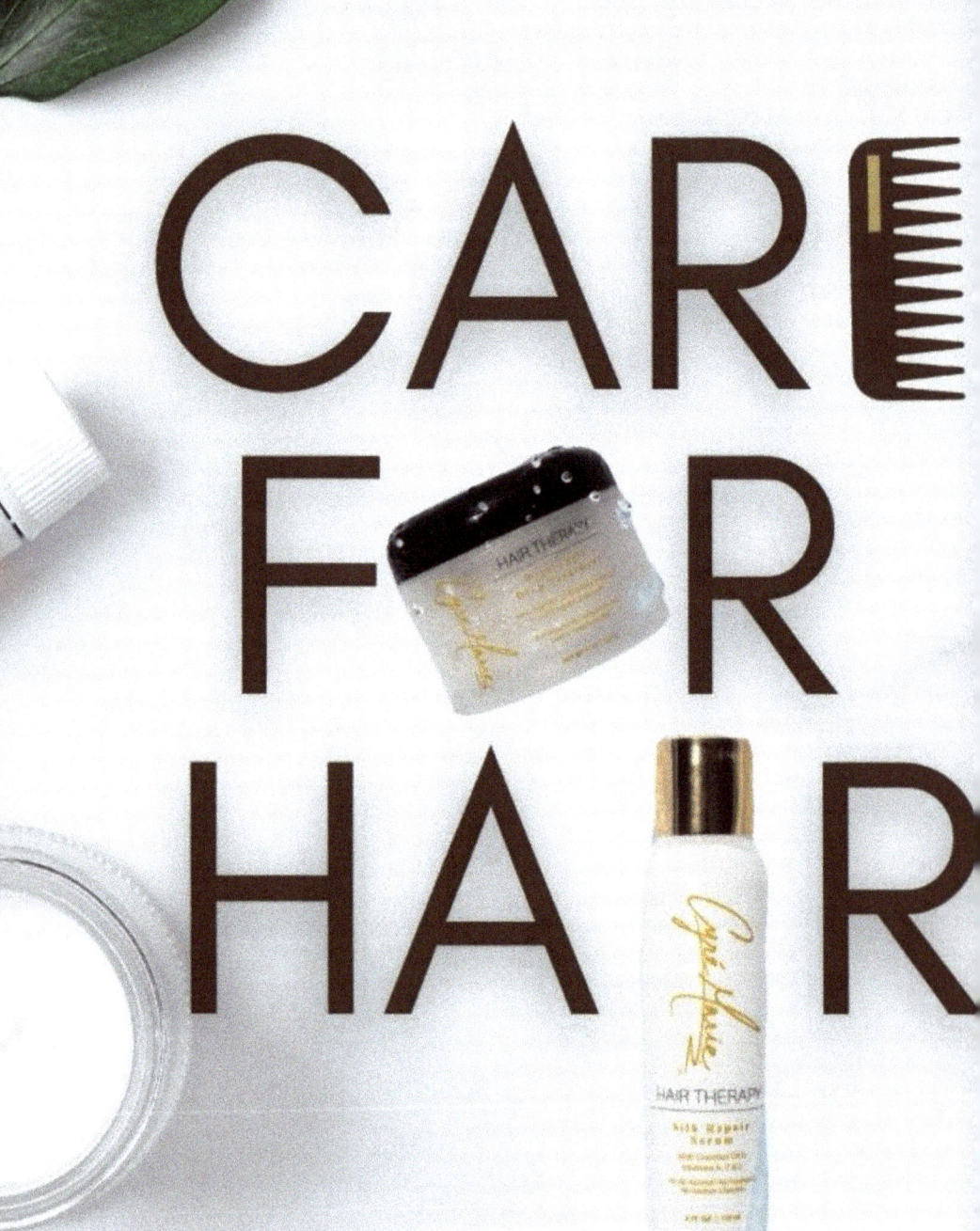

CARE FOR HAIR

Your Ultimate Hair Care Shopping List

Save this list, sis! Whether you're whipping up a deep conditioner, oil blend, or hydration mist, this guide has everything you need to stock up on hair goodies like a pro.

Natural Oils (Sealants & Moisturizers)

- Coconut oil (penetrates the hair shaft)
- Olive oil (adds shine and moisture)
- Argan oil (great for frizz control)
- Jojoba oil (closest to scalp's natural oils)
- Castor oil (promotes hair growth)
- Sweet almond oil (lightweight moisturizer)
- Grapeseed oil (heat protection and shine)
- Avocado oil (deep hydration and nourishment)
- Tea tree oil (scalp clarifying)
- Peppermint oil (stimulates growth)
- Rosemary oil (strengthens and promotes thickness)

Butters & Creams

- Shea butter (locks in moisture)
- Mango butter (lightweight and nourishing)
- Cocoa butter (adds elasticity and softness)

Essential Liquids

- Aloe vera juice (hydration and scalp soothing)
- Apple cider vinegar (scalp detox)
- Rose water (light hydration mist)
- Glycerin (natural humectant for moisture)
- Witch hazel (scalp clarifying)
- Rice water (strengthens hair and adds shine)

DIY Hair Masks Ingredients

- Honey (natural humectant for deep moisture)
- Greek yogurt (protein for strength)
- Eggs (protein-rich treatment)
- Banana (moisture and softness)
- Avocado (deep nourishment)
- Coconut milk (hydrates and repairs)
- Flaxseeds (for DIY hair gel)
- Gelatin powder (for protein treatments)
- Bentonite clay (detoxifying treatment)

Scalp & Hair Treatments

- Tea tree essential oil (anti-dandruff & scalp care)
- Fenugreek seeds (growth and strengthening)
- Black tea (reduces shedding)
- Green tea (stimulates hair follicles)
- Stinging nettle (reduces shedding and promotes growth)

16

Chapter

FEED YOUR FOLLICLES: THE DO'S & DONTS OF HAIR-HEALTHY EATING

VITAMIN MVP
THE REAL HAIR GROWTH SQUAD"

What you put in your body matters just as much as what you put on your hair. Your strands thrive on nutrients, not just deep conditioners and oils. The right foods can fuel growth, shine, and strength– while the wrong ones can leave your hair feeling dull, dry, and prone to breakage.

In this section, we're diving into the do's and don'ts of hair-friendly eating. Because let's be real –no miracle product can outdo a poor diet. Eat smart, and let your hair flourish!

LET'S TALK HAIR BOOSTERS –

Because Magic Ain't Real (But Science Is!)"

Alright, girlfriend, let's keep it real—good hair isn't just about what you put on it, it's about what you put in you. No DIY hair mask in the world can outdo a body that's crying out for nutrients. So, if you're out here drinking soda like it's a green juice and wondering why your hair won't flourish, let's fix that.

Here's your cheat sheet to hair-loving vitamins that can help with growth, thickness, and overall hair health. Take notes, babe.

THE GLOW-UP GANG:
VITAMINS THAT HELP HAIR GROWTH

Biotin (Vitamin B7)

The Beyoncé of hair vitamins. Biotin helps with keratin production, aka the building blocks of your hair. If your strands are feeling weak and shedding like a nervous cat, Biotin is your bestie.

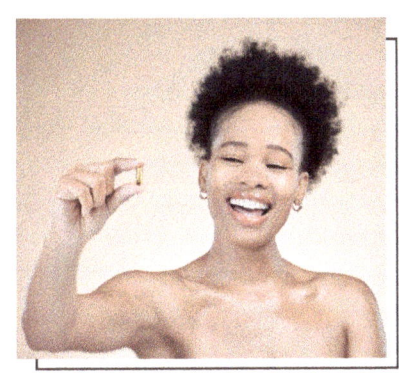

Best time to take

In the morning with food (water-soluble, so it absorbs best this way).

Vitamin D

If your hair is ghosting you (aka thinning or not growing), low Vitamin D could be the problem. A lot of us are deficient and don't even know it!

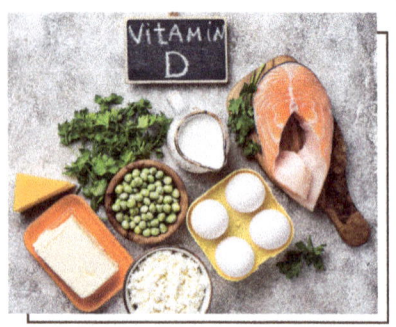

Best time to take
Morning with healthy fats (think avocado toast or eggs).

Iron

Sis, if you're always tired AND your hair is shedding, you might be low on iron. Iron helps your blood deliver oxygen to your hair follicles, and without enough of it, your hair might tap out.

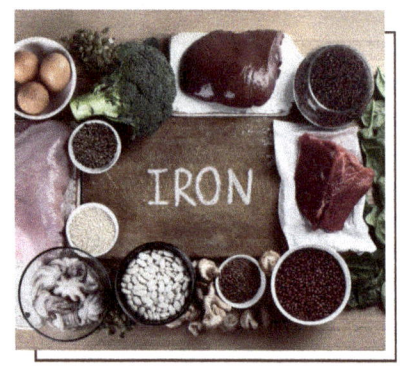

Best time to take
On an empty stomach with Vitamin C (like orange juice) for better absorption.

Omega-3s

Dry, brittle hair? Omega-3s hydrate your scalp from within, keeping your strands soft, shiny, and strong.

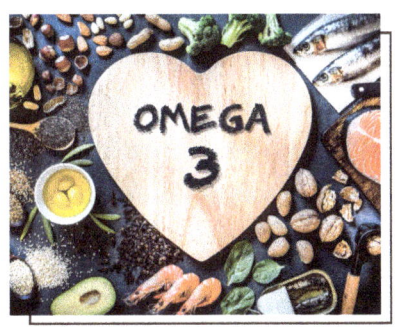

Best time to take
With a meal containing healthy fats (like salmon or avocado).

Collagen & Vitamin C

Think of these two as the dynamic duo for thicker, stronger hair. Collagen supports hair structure, while Vitamin C helps your body absorb it better.

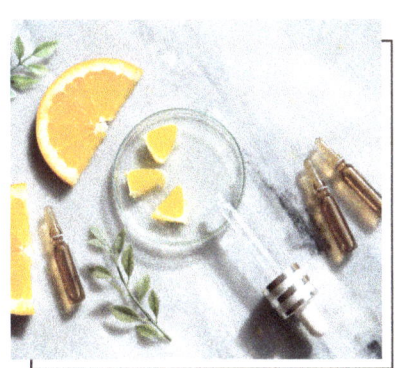

Best time to take
In the morning, mixed in water or your smoothie.

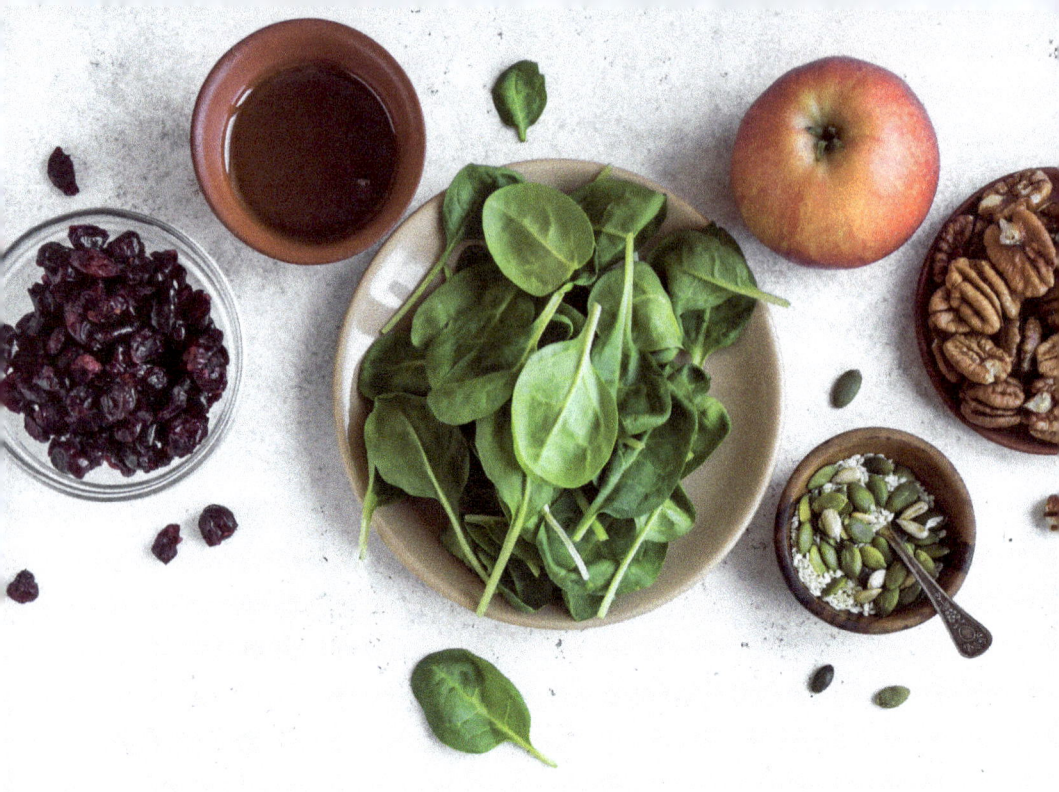

Food for Thought... and Your Edges"

What to eat or Not....

"Feed Your Hair Right"

To get straight to it: if you wouldn't put it in a blender, pour it over your head, or feed it to your plant babies, chances are your hair doesn't want it either. What you eat directly impacts your strands–think of your diet as the VIP treatment your hair deserves.

This section breaks down the do's and don'ts of hair-friendly foods because healthy, thriving hair starts from the inside out. Let's make sure what's on your plate is helping your hair glow, not stunt its shine!

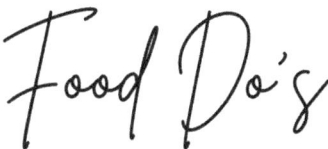

Food Do's

You Are What You Eat (And So Is Your Hair

Here's the breakdown of foods to incorporate for thriving hair and the ones you should kindly leave on the shelf:

The Do's: Foods to Love for Healthy Hair

1. Salmon & Other Fatty Fish
 • Rich in omega-3 fatty acids, which keep your scalp hydrated and hair shiny. Think of it as the natural glow-up for your strands.

2. Eggs
 • Packed with protein and biotin—two major keys for stronger, healthier hair. Skip the supplements; start with brunch!

3. Spinach & Leafy Greens
 • Loaded with iron, which keeps your hair from falling out. Hair loss isn't cute, so eat your greens, sis.

4. Sweet Potatoes
 • Full of beta-carotene (which converts to vitamin A) to help your scalp stay moisturized and your hair grow faster than that one weed in your garden.

5. Nuts & Seeds (Almonds, Walnuts, Flaxseeds)
 • High in zinc, selenium, and healthy fats—aka the ingredients for hair that's snatched, not stressed.

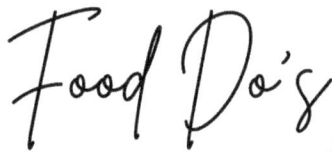

Food Do's

6. Berries
• Packed with antioxidants and vitamin C to protect your hair follicles and boost collagen production. Basically, it's like skincare for your hair.

7. Greek Yogurti
• A great source of protein and vitamin B5 (aka pantothenic acid), which helps prevent thinning hair. Add some honey for sweetness without the guilt.

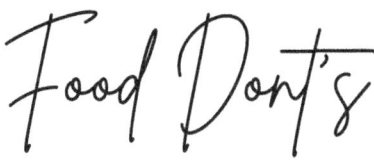

Food Dont's

The Don'ts: Foods to Avoid for Healthy Hair

1. Sugary Snacks & Drinks
• Sugar spikes insulin levels, which can lead to hair thinning and scalp inflammation. That soda? Not worth it, sis.

2. Fast Food (Greasy and Fried)
• Greasy foods clog your pores—including the ones on your scalp. Bye-bye healthy hair growth.

3. Too Much Dairy
• While calcium is great, excess dairy can increase sebum production, leading to dandruff and clogged hair follicles.

4. High-Sodium Foods (Chips, Canned Soups)
• Salt can dehydrate your body—and your hair. Dry, brittle strands are not the look.

5. Alcohol
• Dehydrates your hair and body, leaving your strands dry and lifeless. Maybe skip that extra cocktail?

6. Low-Protein Diets
• Protein is your hair's bestie. Without it, your strands can weaken and break. Don't play your hair like that.

Let's Make This Fun!

This isn't about rules or restrictions—it's about learning, experimenting, and celebrating your hair's journey. Every small win counts, so let's document, track, and celebrate your progress.

Your hair is about to flourish like never before—let's get into it!

CLOSING THOUGHTS:
YOUR HAIR, YOUR CROWN, YOUR JOURNEY

Sis, you made it to the end—but really, this is just the beginning. Your hair journey isn't a one-size-fits-all adventure; it's personal, unique, and ever-evolving. Whether you're deep conditioning like a pro, perfecting your protective styles, or trying out that DIY recipe you've been eyeing—know that every step you take is a step toward healthier, happier hair.

I hope this book has given you the confidence to love your hair in all its glory and the tools to take the best possible care of it. Remember, it's not just about the products you use or the styles you wear—it's about embracing your hair with patience, care, and a whole lot of self-love.

What's Next?

Hair care is a lifelong journey, and I encourage you to:

- Stay Consistent: Your hair loves routine, so stick to what works and tweak as needed.
- Listen to Your Hair: It's always telling you what it needs—pay attention, take notes, and adjust accordingly.
- Celebrate the Wins: Every inch of growth, every successful style, and every small victory is worth celebrating.
- Be Patient: Healthy hair doesn't happen overnight, and that's okay. Enjoy the process.

Let's Stay Connected!

I'd love to hear about your progress, see your results, and connect with you beyond these pages. Let's keep the conversation going:

- Follow me on social media: @Cyre.Marie on IG
- Tag me in your hair journey posts using: #HairTherapyByCM
- Visit my website for more tips, products, and updates.

And hey—if you loved this book, share it with your sisters, friends, and anyone else who needs a little hair love in their life. Let's continue building a community of confident, empowered women who are proud of their crowns.

Final Words:

Your hair is a reflection of you—bold, beautiful, and uniquely yours. Treat it well, love it fiercely, and wear your crown with pride. Until next time, keep thriving and slaying.

With love,

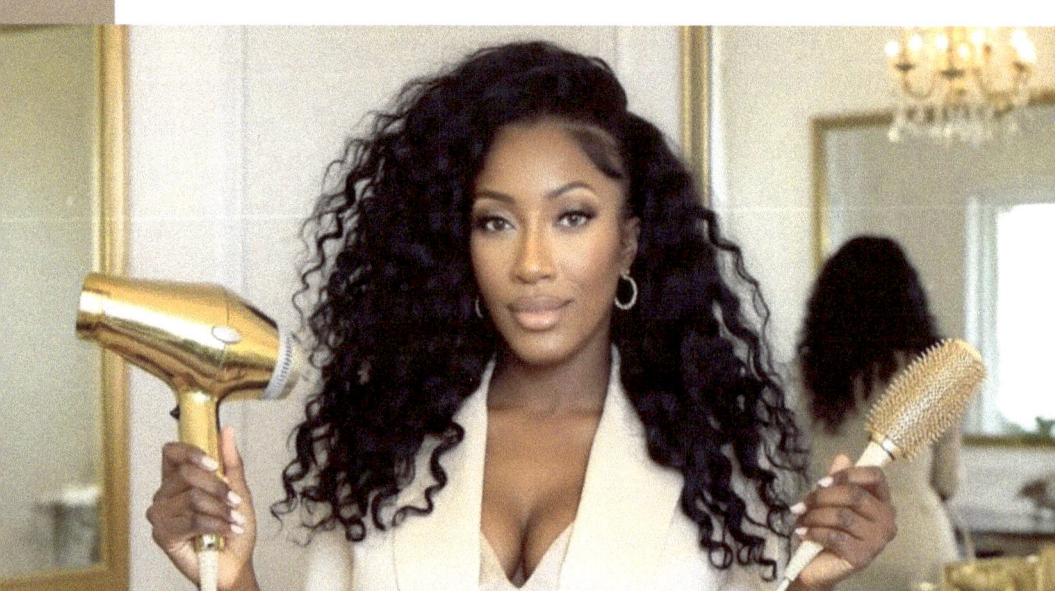

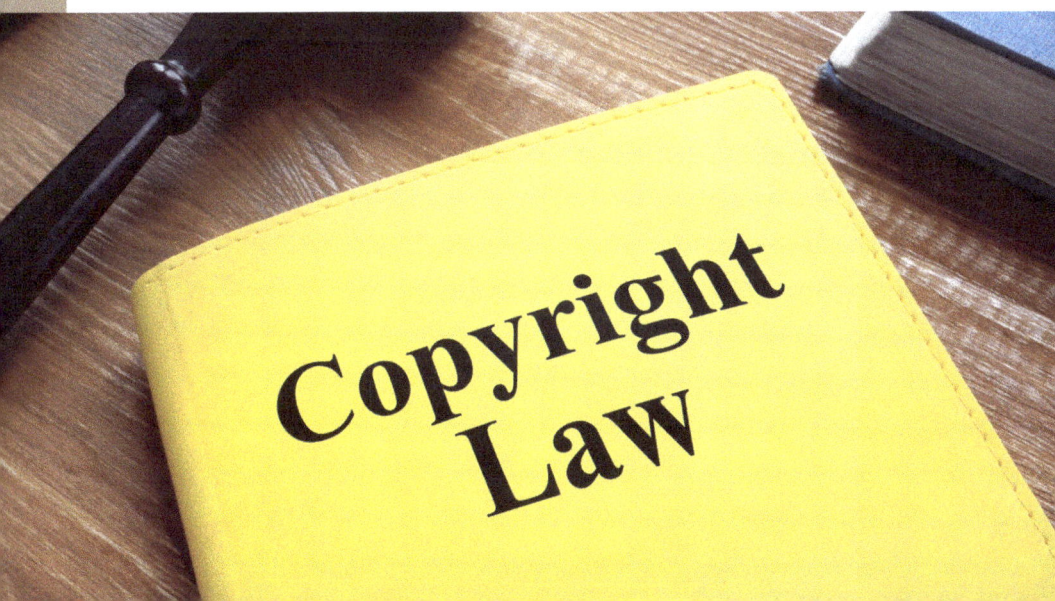

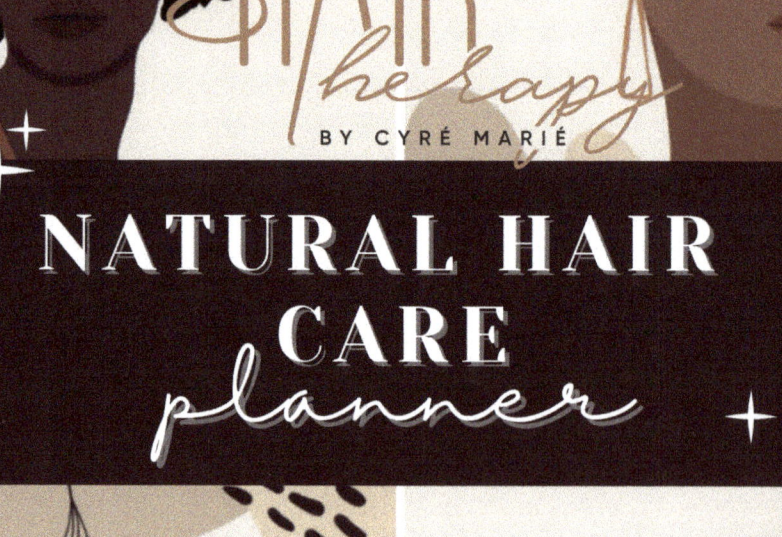

HAIR
Therapy
BY CYRÉ MARIÉ

NATURAL HAIR CARE
planner

BY THE POSITIVE NATURAL

THIS PLANNER BELONGS TO:

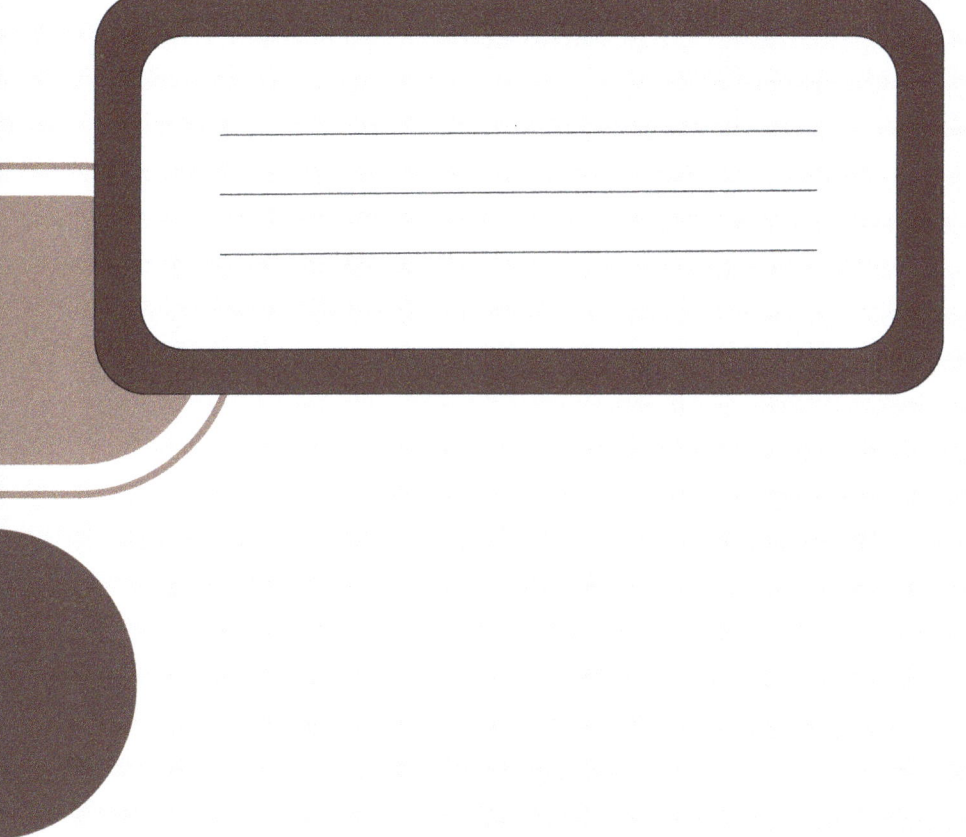

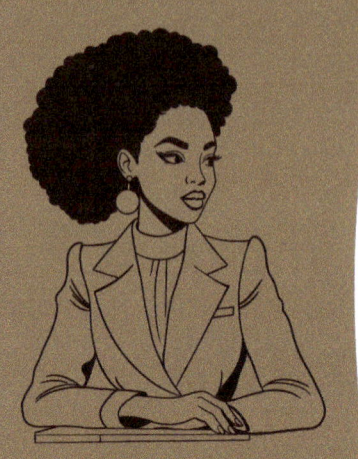

Hey, Gorgeous!

First things first—welcome to your Hair Therapy Journal, your personal space to track, learn, and glow up your hair journey! Whether you're here to grow your curls, maintain silk press perfection, or just figure out what works best for your hair, you've got the right guide in your hands. This isn't just a journal—it's your hair diary, bestie, and accountability partner all in one. So grab your pen (or your favorite stylus), pour up a little self-care tea, and let's get to it.

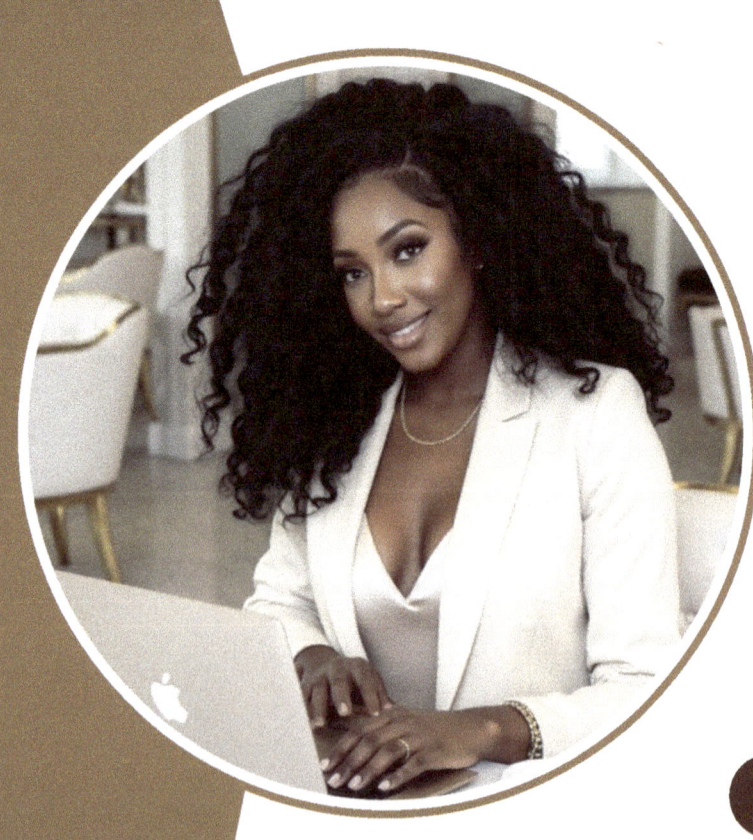

2025 Calendar

JANUARY

S	M	T	W	T	F	S
			1	2	3	4
5	6	7	8	9	10	11
12	13	14	15	16	17	18
19	20	21	22	23	24	25
26	27	28	29	30	31	

FEBRUARY

S	M	T	W	T	F	S
						1
2	3	4	5	6	7	8
9	10	11	12	13	14	15
16	17	18	19	20	21	22
23	24	25	26	27	28	

MARCH

S	M	T	W	T	F	S
						1
2	3	4	5	6	7	8
9	10	11	12	13	14	15
16	17	18	19	20	21	22
23	24	25	26	27	28	29
30	31					

APRIL

S	M	T	W	T	F	S
		1	2	3	4	5
6	7	8	9	10	11	12
13	14	15	16	17	18	19
20	21	22	23	24	25	26
27	28	29	30			

MAY

S	M	T	W	T	F	S
				1	2	3
4	5	6	7	8	9	10
11	12	13	14	15	16	17
18	19	20	21	22	23	24
25	26	27	28	29	30	31

JUNE

S	M	T	W	T	F	S
1	2	3	4	5	6	7
8	9	10	11	12	13	14
15	16	17	18	19	20	21
22	23	24	25	26	27	28
29	30					

JULY

S	M	T	W	T	F	S
		1	2	3	4	5
6	7	8	9	10	11	12
13	14	15	16	17	18	19
20	21	22	23	24	25	26
27	28	29	30	31		

AUGUST

S	M	T	W	T	F	S
					1	2
3	4	5	6	7	8	9
10	11	12	13	14	15	16
17	18	19	20	21	22	23
24	25	26	27	28	29	30
31						

SEPTEMBER

S	M	T	W	T	F	S
	1	2	3	4	5	6
7	8	9	10	11	12	13
14	15	16	17	18	19	20
21	22	23	24	25	26	27
28	29	30				

OCTOBER

S	M	T	W	T	F	S
			1	2	3	4
5	6	7	8	9	10	11
12	13	14	15	16	17	18
19	20	21	22	23	24	25
26	27	28	29	30	31	

NOVEMBER

S	M	T	W	T	F	S
						1
2	3	4	5	6	7	8
9	10	11	12	13	14	15
16	17	18	19	20	21	22
23	24	25	26	27	28	29
30						

DECEMBER

S	M	T	W	T	F	S
	1	2	3	4	5	6
7	8	9	10	11	12	13
14	15	16	17	18	19	20
21	22	23	24	25	26	27
28	29	30	31			

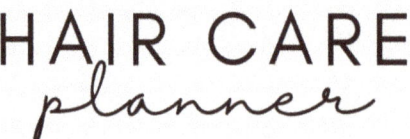

HAIR CARE
planner

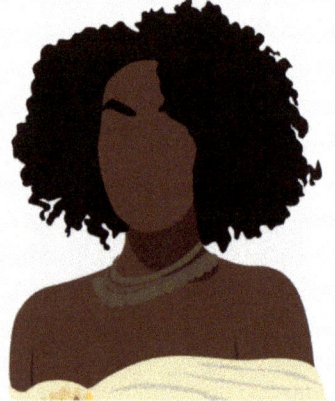

Hair Goals

"I didn't go
natural, I
started to
love the hair I
was born
with."

DO YOU KNOW YOUR
HAIR TYPE?

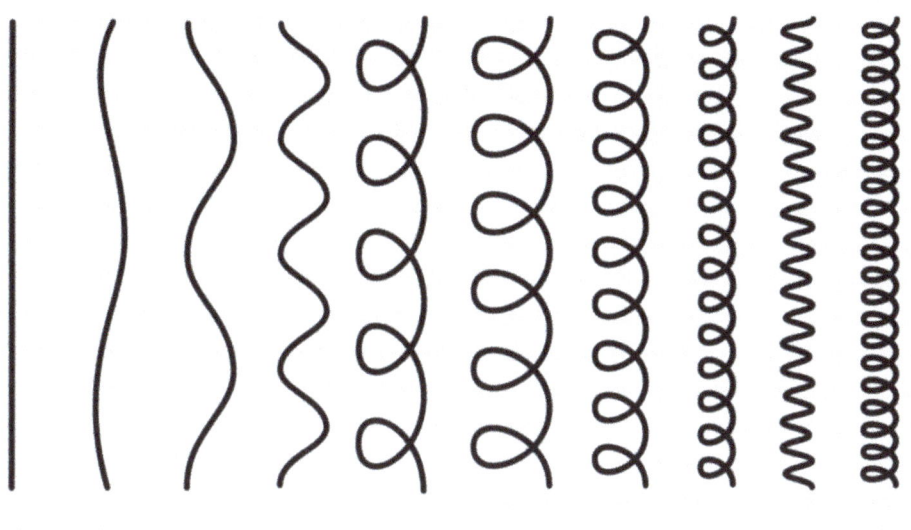

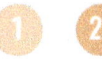 1   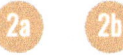 2a   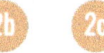 2b   2c   3a   3b   3c   4a   4b   4c

Healthy hair requires an understanding of your hair's porosity, texture, and curl pattern. Knowing your hair type will help you determine how much shampoo to use and even how much heat styling necessary. Products that may work for one type of curly hair may be detrimental to another.

MY HAIR TYPE IS:

DO YOU KNOW YOUR
HAIR POROSITY?

LOW
POROSITY

MEDIUM
POROSITY

HIGH
POROSITY

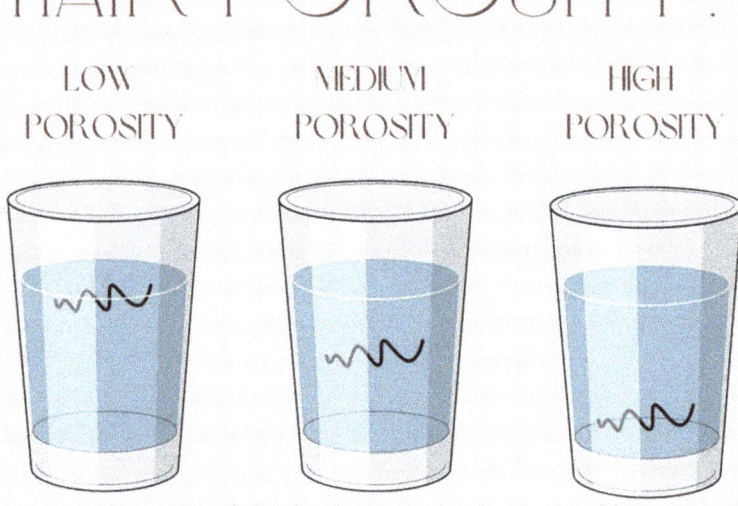

The tight, protective cuticle of the hair must be penetrated by water, oils, and other moisturizing agents in order to reach the cortex and maintain the health of the hair. However, that isn't always easy to do in hair with low or high porosity. In low porosity conditions, the cuticles may be excessively close together, making it difficult for hair to receive the moisture it needs. Hair may not be able to retain moisture in high porosity situations because of the overly split cuticles.

There are three different types of hair porosity.

- **Low Porosity**
  - The cuticles of hair with low porosity are closely spaced. Moisture finds it challenging to enter the hair shaft as a result.
- **Medium Porosity**
  - Hair with a medium porosity has less firmly bonded cuticles. This implies that moisture can permeate your hair more quickly and stay in your hair for a longer amount of time.
- **High Porosity**
  - The cuticles of hair with high porosity are more widely spaced. Although the hair can readily absorb moisture, it cannot do so for an extended period of time. Due to genetics or hair damage, the cuticles have gaps between them.

DO YOU KNOW YOUR
HAIR POROSITY?

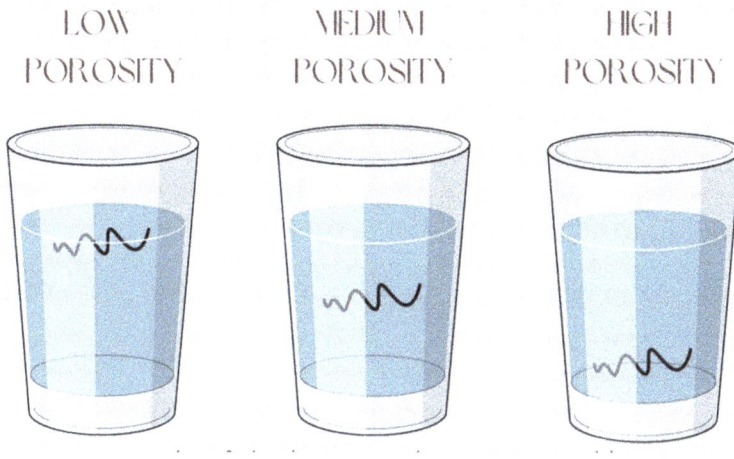

LOW POROSITY

MEDIUM POROSITY

HIGH POROSITY

HOW TO DETERMINE HAIR POROSITY

Here's an easy test for hair porosity.

1. *Shampoo and rinse your hair. This step is critical to remove any product buildup. Wait until your hair is dry.*
2. *Fill a glass with water. Dip a single strand of hair into the glass of water.*
3. *Watch the strand to see if it sinks or floats. You can determine your hair's porosity from the results.*

- Low porosity = The strand floats at the top before sinking
- Medium porosity = The strand floats somewhere in the middle of the glass
- High porosity = The strand quickly sinks to the bottom of the glass

You may also check the porosity of your hair by simply sliding your finger down a strand of your hair, you may check the porosity of your hair. You might not be able to tell as easily because this test is more objective. Because the cuticles are open, hair with low porosity will feel smooth, whereas hair with high porosity would feel rough. The determination of medium porosity hair with this method is more challenging, though.

Hair Properties

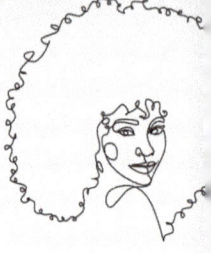

HAIR HEALTH

Heat Damage	♡	♡	♡	♡	♡
Chemical Damge	♡	♡	♡	♡	♡
Moisture	♡	♡	♡	♡	♡
Ends	♡	♡	♡	♡	♡
Edges	♡	♡	♡	♡	♡

PROPERTIES

Texture:

Porosity:

Elasticity:

Density:

GOAL SETTING

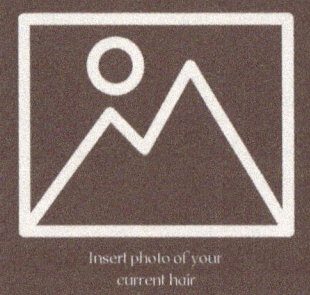

Insert photo of your
current hair

Current Length:

Notes:

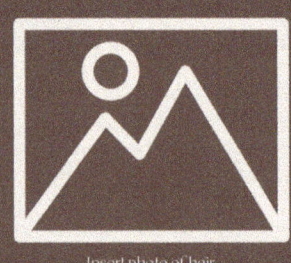

Insert photo of hair
inspiration or goal

Desired Length:

Goals:

NOTES

....

....

....

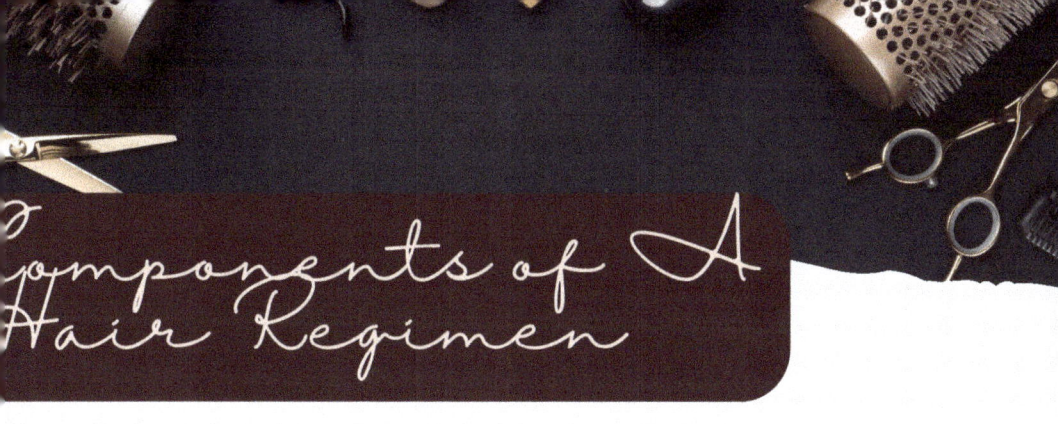

Components of A Hair Regimen

CLEANSING

- Cleaning is a crucial step in your natural hair care routine. This is where you get rid of the buildup on your scalp and hair. This is an essential component of any regimen if you want your hair to keep growing.
- Instead of just co-washing, use an all-natural, hydrating shampoo that is sulfate-free. It is your choice how often you decide to wash your hair. Most people who have natural hair wash it once every week to once a month. You can experiment with this frequency to determine what works best for you.

CONDITIONING

- Rinse-out or daily conditioner: You can use a daily conditioner any time you wet your hair. It is meant to be washed out, as opposed to a leave-in conditioner. Your hair becomes more hydrated, which also helps with detangling. If you battle with frizz, it also makes it less likely to occur.
- Leave-in conditioner: After washing your hair, you can refill and maintain moisture using a thin leave-in conditioner. After washing and before styling, it is suggested that you use a leave-in conditioner on moist hair. With leave-in, you don't have to be too frugal - you can use it all the time!
- Deep conditioner: This conditioner is applied to the hair and allowed to sit in the hair for a predetermined amount of time before being rinsed away. Compared to the other types, this conditioner isn't used as frequently. In fact, others have likened it to a "five-star meal." It has a ton of nutrients and moisture that aid in detangling, softening, and many other processes. For maximum benefits, thorough conditioning should only be done once every two weeks or so.

MOISTURIZING

- It's likely that moisture (or lack of it) is the cause of hair loss, breakage, dryness, tangling, or matting. Your hair's porosity will determine how much moisture you require. However, everyday hydration (focused on the ends) is required by the majority of naturals.
- Hydrate your hair before bed and wrap it in a silk scarf or pillowcase at night to keep it as moist as possible. Additionally, you can moisten during the day using the LOC technique, steam, or a refresher spray.

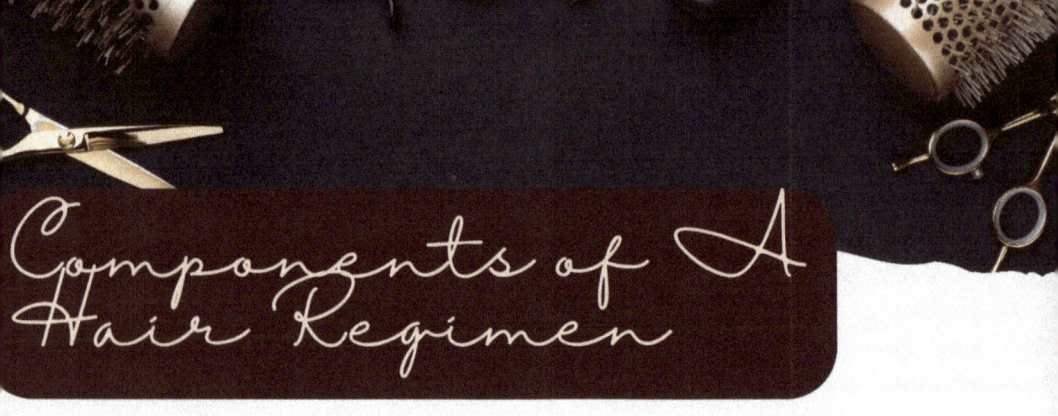

Components of A Hair Regimen

SEALING

- You should be aware of how crucial moisture is to healthy hair. But for it to stay, you must seal the moisture in. To keep your hair hydrated throughout the day, try using a sealer or anti-humectant.
- Recommendations based on hair type:
  - Coarser or thicker hair: shea butter or Jamaican black castor oil
  - Finer hair: olive oil, jojoba oil, or avocado oil

DETANGLING

- As it lowers hair loss, matting, dryness, and breakage, detangling should be a frequent component of your hair routine. A curly girl may detest detangling, but the more you do it, the less difficult it will become. Here is how the procedure ought to go.
  - On moist hair, use a wide-tooth comb.
  - Pull down from the ends first, then ascend beginning at the top. This decreases breakage.
  - Add a leave-in conditioner to the hair if detangling is especially challenging, or detangle while running your hair under warm water.

STYLING & PROTECTING

- Protective styling must be a part of a hair regimen to encourage growth. Any style that minimizes combing or other manipulation of the hair is considered protective. It prevents heat from being used, keeps your hair up and away from your shoulders. For instance, protective hairstyles like twist-outs, buns, spiral curls, and braids are common.

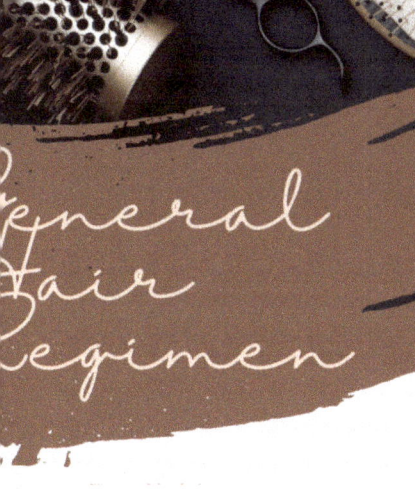

General Hair Regimen

DAILY

- mist hair with water or daily spray
- scalp massage
- re-twist at night
- protect hair with satin scarf or bonnet
- sleep with silk pillowcase

MID-WEEK

- moisturize
- LCO or LOC method
- apply oil and butters
- oil and massage scalp

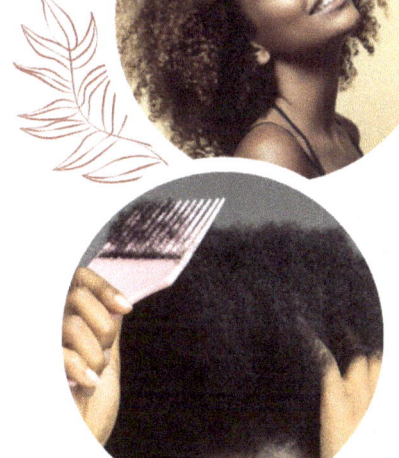

WEEKLY

- wash day routine or co-wash
- pre-poo
- detangle
- deep condition
- low manipulation styles
- protective styles
- diy treatments or hair masks

MONTHLY

- protein treatment
- clay mask
- clarifying treatment
- scalp detox

Trim your ends quarterly or every 3-6 months

BUILD YOUR OWN HAIR REGIMEN

DAILY

WEEKLY

MONTHLY

DAILY PLAN

DATE

TODAY'S HAIR TO-DO'S

- [ ]
- [ ]
- [ ]
- [ ]
- [ ]
- [ ]
- [ ]
- [ ]
- [ ]
- [ ]

AFFIRMATION OF THE DAY

DAILY QUOTE

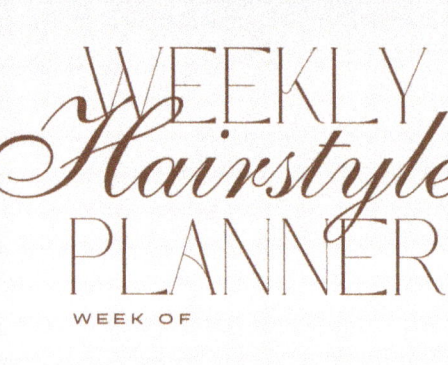

WEEKLY
Hairstyle
PLANNER

WEEK OF

Monday

Tuesday

Wednesday

Thursday

Friday

Saturday

Sunday

Wash Day Timeline

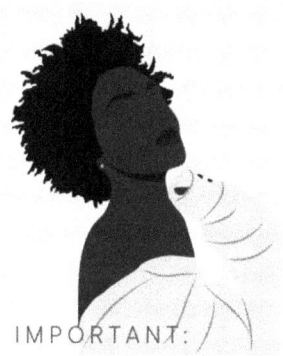

WEEK OF:

HAIRSTYLE
:

IMPORTANT:

STEP 1
STEP 2
STEP 3
STEP 4
STEP 5
STEP 6
STEP 7

NOTES:

Monthly

HAIR PLANS

JAN	FEB	MAR	APR	MAY	JUN
JUL	AUG	SEP	OCT	NOV	DEC

Sunday	Monday	Tuesday	Wednesday	Thursday	Friday	Saturday

notes

MONTHLY HAIR CHECK-IN

FAVORITE PRODUCTS

JOURNAL

How has my natural hair improved?

How has the way I feel and speak about my natural hair improved?

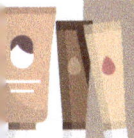

HAIR HEALTH

What To Avoid	What Helps

NATURAL HAIR
Affirmations

- The love and care I put into my hair is paying off.
- I have a hair routine that is custom to my hair type and needs.
- I am learning to love my hair more and more every day.
- I take advantage of the resources that educate me on proper hair care.
- I choose to be patient with myself as I learn proper haircare techniques.
- When I wear my natural hair, I feel beautiful, unique, and authentic.
- I love seeing my natural hair grow and glow.
- I am blessed to have the hair that I do. My strands are full of history and strength.
- My hair is becoming healthier everyday.
- I speak positively about my hair texture.
- I am an artist and my hair is the canvas.
- No mistakes were made on me or my hair texture.
- My hair is naturally beautiful and strong.
- I am confident in my curls.
- I am worthy of the time I spend on my hair and self care.
- My hair is my crown and I wear it with pride.

CREATE YOUR
OWN HAIR
Affirmations

_____

_____

_____

_____

_____

_____

_____

_____

_____

_____

_____

_____

_____

_____

CREATE YOUR
OWN HAIR
Affirmations

CREATE YOUR
OWN HAIR
Affirmations

GOAL TRACKER

JANUARY

FEBRUARY

MARCH

APRIL

MAY

JUNE

GOAL TRACKER

JULY

AUGUST

SEPTEMBER

OCTOBER

NOVEMBER

DECEMBER

FIVE GREAT HAIR OILS & THEIR BENEFITS

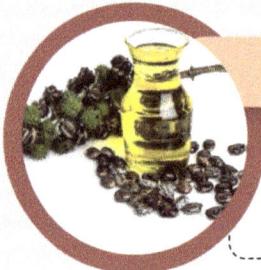

CASTOR OIL

seals moisture, promotes hair growth, & improves scalp health

AVOCADO OIL

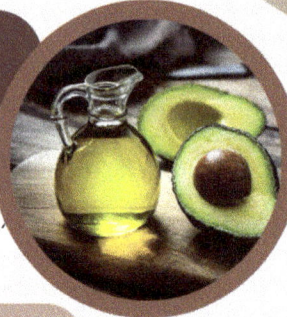

prevents damage & promotes healthy cell growth

OLIVE OIL

promotes scalp health, circulation, & stimulates growth for thicker hair

ALMOND OIL

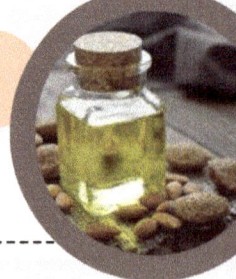

treats dandruff, reduces inflammation, & improves circulation

JOJOBA OIL

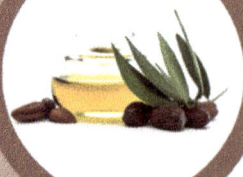

removes build up and frizz, reduces dry scalp & irritation

TIPS TO ACHIEVE AND MAINTAIN HAIR GROWTH

- **Maintain a healthy diet**
  - A balanced diet is critical for general health just as it is for the growth of your natural hair
- **Learn what hair products and habits work for your hair type**
  - All curl types require moisture and hydration, regardless of whether you have low or high porosity hair. It's important to get the greatest natural hair products for growth, but not all products are one-size-fits-all
- **Drink plenty of water**
  - Natural hair constantly craves moisture, so stay hydrated to nourish your strands from the inside out to achieve optimal hair growth
- **Protect your hair at night**
  - Wear a satin scarf or bonnet or sleep on a satin pillow case to maintain hydration and retain moisture
- **Get trims regularly**
  - Trimming your hair helps to get rid of damaged, broken, or split ends
- **Moisturize and massage the scalp**
  - Scalp massages are a fantastic way to improve blood flow to the hair follicles and spur hair growth
- **Avoid tight or high-manipulation hairstyles**
  - Tight hairstyles can often pull at the roots or cause breakage which can make it harder to retain length
- **Take your vitamins and/or supplements**
  - A hair, skin, and nails vitamin is a great option for growing natural hair

HAIR RECIPES

INGREDIENTS

....

....

....

....

....

....

....

....

....

Prep Time:

Application Time:

Rating:

☆☆☆☆☆

STEPS

_____

_____

_____

_____

_____

HAIR RECIPES

INGREDIENTS

....

....

....

....

....

....

....

....

....

....

Prep Time:

Application Time:

Rating:

☆☆☆☆☆

STEPS

HAIR RECIPES

INGREDIENTS

....
....
....
....
....
....
....
....
....

Prep Time:

Application Time:

Rating:

☆☆☆☆☆

STEPS

_____
_____
_____
_____
_____

HAIR RECIPES

INGREDIENTS

....

....

....

....

....

....

....

....

....

Prep Time:

Application Time:

Rating:

☆☆☆☆☆

STEPS

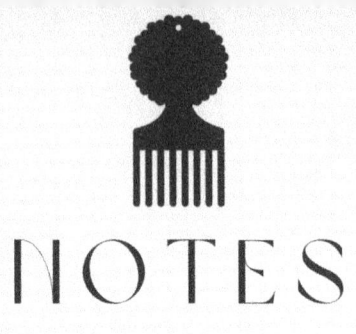

NOTES

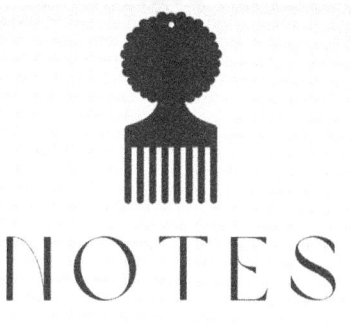

NOTES

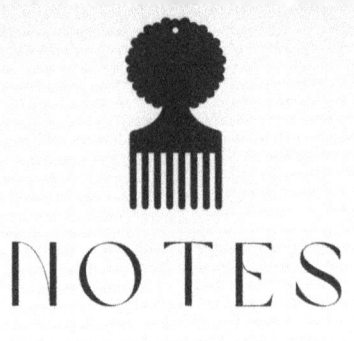

NOTES

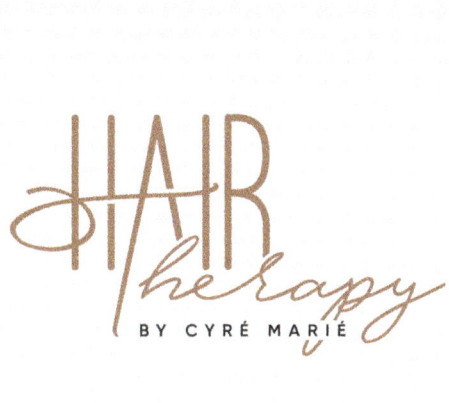

Thank You for Being a Part of Hair Therapy!

our hair journey is your story, and we're honored to be a part of it. Whether you're here for growth, hydration, or just a little extra self-care, remember—healthy hair is a commitment, and you deserve to feel confident every step of the way.

f you loved this guide, let's stay connected! Follow Hair herapy on Instagram, TikTok, Pinterest, and YouTube for more tips, recipes, and inspiration.

Here's to strong strands, flourishing curls, and a journey ' with love and self-care! Keep in touch. Follow me ram @Cyre.Marie & @Hairtherapy.cm on YouTube search Cyre Marie

Hello@CyreMarie.com
CyreMarie.com

www.ingramcontent.com/pod-product-compliance
Lightning Source LLC
Chambersburg PA
CBHW051514120626
46551CB00012B/916